PROFESSIONAL TURNOVER:
The Case of Nurses

Health Systems Management
Series editor, **Samuel Levey, Ph.D.,** University of Iowa

Volume 1:
Financial Management of Health Institutions
J. B. Silvers and C. K. Prahalad 1974

Volume 2:
Personnel Administration in the Health Services Industry: Theory and Practice, 2nd ed.
Norman Metzger 1979

Volume 3:
The National Labor Relations Act: A Guidebook for Health Care Facility Administrators
Dennis D. Pointer and Norman Metzger 1975

Volume 4:
Organizational Issues in Health Care Management
Alan Sheldon 1975

Volume 5:
Long Term Care: A Handbook for Researchers, Planners and Providers
Edited by Sylvia Sherwood 1975

Volume 6:
Analysis of Urban Health Problems: Case Studies from the Health Services Administration of the City of New York
Edited by Irving Leveson and Jeffrey H. Weiss 1976

Volume 7:
Health Maintenance Organizations: A Guide to Planning and Development
Roger W. Birnbaum 1976

Volume 8:
Labor Arbitration in Health Care
Edited by Earl R. Baderschneider and Paul F. Miller 1976

Volume 9:
The Consumer and the Health Care System: Social and Managerial Perspectives
Edited by Harry Rosen, Jonathan M. Metsch and Samuel Levey 1977

Volume 10:
Long-Term Care Administration: A Managerial Perspective, I & II
Edited by Samuel Levey and N. Paul Loomba 1977

Volume 11:
Hospital Organization and Management: Text and Readings, 2nd ed.
Edited by Jonathon S. Rakich and Kurt Darr 1978

Volume 12:
Democratic Processes for Modern Health Agencies
Irving Ladimer with Joel C. Solomon and Stanley G. House 1979

Volume 13:
Curing and Caring: A Review of the Factors Affecting the Quality and Acceptability of Health Care
Allen D. Spiegel and Bernard Backhaut 1980

Volume 14:
Evaluation Concepts and Methods: Shaping Policy for the Health Administrator
Paul C. Nutt 1981

Volume 15:
Professional Turnover: The Case of Nurses
James L. Price and Charles W. Mueller 1981

PROFESSIONAL TURNOVER: The Case of Nurses

James L. Price
and
Charles W. Mueller
Department of Sociology
University of Iowa
Iowa City, Iowa

SP MEDICAL & SCIENTIFIC BOOKS
New York

Dedication

To Lee and Anna Mary

Softcover reprint of the hardcover 1st edition 1981

SPECTRUM PUBLICATIONS, INC.
175-20 Wexford Terrace, Jamaica, N.Y. 11432

Library of Congress Cataloging in Publication Data

Price, James L
Professional turnover.

(Health systems management series)
Bibliography
Includes index.
1. Nurses—Employment—United States. 2. Hospitals —United States—Staff. 3. Labor turnover—United States. I. Mueller, Charles W., joint author. II. Title. [DNLM: 1. Nurses—Supply and distribution —United States. W1 HE588F v. 15 / WY31 P945p]
RT86.73.P74 331.12'6 80-11553
ISBN 978-94-011-8018-4 ISBN 978-94-011-8016-0 (eBook)
DOI 10.1007/978-94-011-8016-0

Acknowledgments

We would like to thank the Division of Nursing, Bureau of Health Manpower (RO2-NU-00593) and the American Nurses' Foundation for funds to perform this research. The difficult role of patron was admirably fulfilled by these organizations. Dr. Myrtle K. Aydelotte (Executive Director, American Nurses' Association, and Professor, College of Nursing, University of Iowa) greatly encouraged us when we were most in need of support. Her tangible assistance is very much appreciated.

Although intellectually stimulating, data collection for field research is a constant source of anxiety, even with the most cooperative respondents. Our anxiety was kept at the minimum level by the extraordinary cooperation of the employees in the seven hospitals we studied; they were ideal respondents. We extend our heartfelt thanks to them and hope that our research will be of some assistance to them in the performance of their work.

We continue to be amazed at the number of editorial improvements that Ben Haller can make on the "final" copies that we turn in to him. His keen editorial judgments were very helpful. The task of translating our rough drafts and rewrites into legible typed pages was given to Gail Chadwick. The speed and precision with which she completed this task was remarkable and never allowed us the opportunity to "blame the typist" for our not meeting deadlines.

Quality research assistants are a vital ingredient of a first-rate university program of scholarship. We were fortunate to have had three such assistants during the course of our project: Mark Dickson, James Curry, and William Montgomery. When our funds were depleted, Ron Akers (Chairman, Department of Sociology, University of Iowa) generously continued to provide financial support for our research assistants.

And last but not least, we would like to thank our many colleagues who have read and criticized various parts of this manuscript. To single out for praise any single colleague is to risk offending others. We must, however especially thank Allen Bluedorn, Arthur Brief, Dan Farrell, Michael Lewis-Beck, Thomas Martin, Gerald Rose, and Robert Szafran. Since we listened to but did not always take their advice, we naturally accept the consequences of our action and take full responsibility for the final product.

Contents

CHAPTER 1
The Problem

The high turnover rate of hospital nurses is well known. Two studies by the American Nurses' Association (1954, 1962) indicate the magnitude of this turnover. A national sample of 311 nonfederal general hospitals conducted in 1954 finds a crude turnover rate of 42 percent among the nurses [1]. A second national sample of 428 nonfederal hospitals, performed in 1962, notes a crude turnover rate of 58 percent among the nurses. Nurses in these two studies thus have an average turnover rate of 50 percent.

Studies of teachers and social workers provide a basis of comparison for the turnover of the nurses. Such comparisons are reasonable because teachers and social workers, like nurses, have about the same amount of educational preparation and are mostly female. Two studies of teachers (Mason and Bain 1959; Lindenfeld 1963) are relevant. A national sample of 1,551 school districts in 1957-1958 finds that the elementary and secondary teachers have a crude turnover rate of 17 percent. A comparable study, conducted in 1959-1960 on 2,179 school districts, indicates a rate of 13 percent among teachers.

Two studies of social workers (Tollen 1960; U.S. Children's Bureau 1965) provide comparable data. A 1957 study of 427 child-welfare and family-service organizations notes that the social workers in the organizations had a crude turnover rate of 34 percent. A figure of 30 percent is reported for the social workers in a 1964 study of 171 state and local welfare organizations.

Hospital nurses, therefore, have more than three times the turnover rate of teachers and more than one and a half times the turnover rate of social workers. Hughes, an eminent occupational sociologist, notes (1958, p. 69) that hospitals are "one of the institutions where many pass through and a few stay on." Nurses, it seems, are hospital employees who more readily "pass through" than "stay on" [2].

Our major objective in this book is to explain the turnover of hospital nurses. The basis of this explanation is a "causal model" developed from a review of the turnover literature. Before this model is described, however, the meaning and significance of turnover must be indicated.

THE MEANING OF TURNOVER

Turnover is voluntary separation of an individual from an organization[3]. "Quits" is probably the most common label used to designate voluntary separations. In this study no attempt will be made to explain involuntary separations, such as dismissals, layoffs, retirements, and deaths. Nor will any effort be made to explain why individuals decide to begin work in organizations. Transfers and promotions, since they take place within organizational boundaries, are also excluded. This research, then, like most research on turnover, focuses only on voluntary separations.

Voluntary separations are most commonly studied because of their frequency and the possibility of control by the organization. Most turnover is voluntary (Price 1977, p. 9). In this research, for example, 20 percent of the nurses left during the approximately fourteen-month period of data collection. Only 1 percent of these nurses, however, left involuntarily—for dismissals, layoffs, retirements, and deaths. Managers also have more control over voluntary separations. Dismissals are generally subject to considerable managerial control, but layoffs, retirements, and deaths are much less manageable.

The focus on voluntary separations does not mean that the nurses who remain in hospital employment will be ignored. As a later chapter on data and methods (Chapter 3) will indicate, our research will classify the sample of nurses into "leavers" and "stayers." The basic task of the analysis will be to see if the leavers and stayers differ significantly on the variables thought to produce variations in turnover. We assume that differing amounts of the same variable have an impact on leavers and stayers. For example, low pay is believed, all other things being equal, to be an important variable producing leavers from organizations, whereas high pay is thought to produce stayers. Our focus on "quits" thus does not mean that "stays" will be ignored. This point requires emphasis because the customary way of stating the problem—stating that our dependent variable is voluntary separation—sometimes conveys the false impression that we will study only leavers. (To simplify our presentation, "turnover" will henceforth be substituted for "voluntary separation.")

SIGNIFICANCE OF HIGH TURNOVER AMONG HOSPITAL NURSES[4]

The significance of high nursing turnover can be examined from the perspective of different units—hospital, society, nursing profession, patients, and so forth. Since the focus of this book is on nursing turnover from hospitals, the significance of turnover will initially be examined from the perspective of the hospital and then from a more general perspective.

Hospital Perspective

There are at least three reasons why high nursing turnover is important to hospitals.

(1) High nursing turnover seriously complicates the hospital's goal of providing quality care for its patients. Nurses are critically important to the hospital because they are the most highly trained professionals whose presence in the hospital is continuous. Physicians, the most highly trained professionals in the hospital, spend very little time in the hospital visiting their patients, and licensed practical nurses, who spend the most time with the patients, have limited professional training. Since nurses

are such a critically important group, and since job performance generally improves with experience, it is desirable to have a large core of experienced nurses in each nursing unit for the day, evening, and night shifts. With a crude turnover rate of approximately 50 percent, such a staffing pattern is impossible to achieve. The experienced nurses must be spread very thinly among the nursing units, thereby complicating the task of providing patient care. Nursing turnover, in short, threatens hospital effectiveness [5].

Not only is the provision of quality patient care threatened by high nursing turnover, but the care that is provided becomes very expensive to maintain. Melbin and Taub (1966), in a careful study of turnover among nurses in a large metropolitan general hospital, estimate that a minimum cost of about $420 was incurred to replace each nurse who left. Since Melbin and Taub's figures pertain to 1965, contemporary costs will, of course, be significantly higher. It is clear that the high rate of nursing turnover is costly to hospitals. If hospitals could significantly reduce their nursing turnover while maintaining existing standards of patient care, then hospital productivity would be noticeably improved [6].

All nursing turnover is, of course, not detrimental to hospital effectiveness. High nursing turnover, for instance, probably makes it easier for hospitals to introduce change because traditional operating procedures are weakened by the movement of employees into and out of hospitals, and in an environment of rapidly changing health-care technology, such as exists in contemporary American society, the quality of patient care is likely to be improved by many of these changes. Nor is all nursing turnover necessarily destructive to productivity. When relatively incompetent nurses leave, for example, costs are likely to be reduced—and patient care improved. The main body of the turnover literature, nevertheless, has focused on the negative impact of turnover on effectiveness and productivity, thereby ignoring possible benefits of turnover for the organization[7]. Our belief, however, which we cannot empirically support in a rigorous fashion, is that when nursing turnover approximates 50 percent, its net effect on effectiveness and productivity is probably negative. The negative effects must, of course, be subtracted from the positive effects to arrive at the net effects.

(2) Hospitals have been urged by scholars to establish "alternate career structures" for nurses[8]. The traditional career structure for hospital nurses usually consists of the following series of ranked occupations: staff nurse, unit supervisor, assistant nursing director, and nursing director. A key characteristic of this traditional structure is that it mostly consists of administrative occupations. Only the beginning occupation—the staff nurse—is primarily a professional occupation.

The traditional career structure seems to have a number of undesirable results. Nurses with little competence in administration often seek to be unit supervisors since this is the only route to increased rewards (money, prestige, and power) within the hospital. Unfortunately, many of these nurses are more competent as nurses than as administrators. In this way the traditional career structure often results in less than competent administration and nursing supervision.

It is also believed that the traditional structure produces turnover. A nurse who wishes to remain a nurse, and who continues to perform in this capacity for many years, soon finds herself/himself at the top of the reward structure. Since few additional rewards are possible in this position, the nurse is motivated to leave the hospital, and probably the profession. The traditional career structure is probably one reason why one observes few older nurses in hospitals.

An alternate career structure would establish a series of ranked occupations, all of which primarily involve nursing duties. The occupations might be labeled numerically, as for example, $nurse_1$ through $nurse_4$. As is customary with career structures, the ranking would be in terms of money, prestige, and power: the higher the rank, the greater the reward. With such a structure, some of the $nurse_4$'s would receive more money than some of the nurse supervisors. To move from $nurse_1$ to $nurse_4$ would require only increased competence as a nurse. The baccalaureate nurse, for instance, would not have to leave the hospital to obtain an M.A. degree in administration (or any other course of study) to move to the top of the nursing hierarchy. The alternate career structure would thus seem to correct some of the defects of the traditional career structure and, in the long run, improve nursing performance and the quality of patient care.

Hospitals, however, are reluctant to establish alternate career structures with the high turnover rate of their nurses. Such a structure, for example, requires the investment of sizable hospital resources in training over a long period of time. It requires a large number of training institutes, in-service sessions, weekend conferences, books, journals, and nursing courses to transform an inexperienced $nurse_1$ into an experienced $nurse_4$. If a hospital makes such an investment in its nurses, and if the nurse leaves after the training is complete or near the end of the training, then the hospital does not receive the full benefit of its investment. Hospitals cannot invest their scarce resources in this manner. The irony is that the traditional career structure is probably one source of the turnover that makes it very difficult for hospitals to implement an alternate career structure which would, in turn, help hospitals reduce nursing turnover.

Alternate career structures take on added significance in the context of the changing role of women in American society. In the future, more nurses will probably want to spend more time as nurses, and to accommodate this demand, alternate career structures will be very helpful. More nurses will likely remain single—thus continued work will be a necessity. Nurses who marry and have children increasingly expect to continue in their profession to fulfill themselves and to increase the family income. Finally, nurses who are divorced or separated and who have children commonly continue working as heads of single-parent families. Nurses who spend more of their lives as nurses will require more rewards than the traditional career structure can provide. The reluctance of hospitals to establish alternate career structures for their nurses is likely to result in serious long-term problems in the management of hospitals, given these trends in American society.

(3) Concern is often expressed about the geographical maldistribution of nurses in the United States. Some areas of the country, especially the large cities, seem to have an adequate supply of the available nurses. Although many cities have experienced shortages of nurses, the shortages in rural areas and small communities are even more serious. Highly trained professionals, such as nurses, seem to prefer the large cities. The maldistribution is made even more serious because most nursing education is financed by the states rather than by the federal government. The state of Iowa, for instance, is not too happy to use its limited financial resources to train nurses who promptly leave the state when their training is complete. Iowa, of course, receives some nurses from other states, but more seem to leave than come in.

The geographical maldistribution of nurses is, of course, part of a general problem, the maldistribution of all types of health-care professionals. And the problem is not limited to the United States but characterizes all modern, and modernizing, countries. Solution of the problem is very complex. New types of nurses and physicians may have to be trained and new types of social arrangements may have to be established to begin to solve this problem. The point we wish to make is that high nursing turnover complicates the solution of this problem. If some type of hospital continues to service small communities and rural areas, and if these hospitals can in some way recruit sufficient nurses to staff their positions, then turnover of these nurses—many of whom will migrate to the large cities—undermines all the efforts to distribute nurses more evenly throughout the United States. It does little good to recruit nurses to staff hospitals in rural areas and small communities if the nurses do not remain in the hospitals. Without a lowering of the turnover rate of hospital nurses, it will be very difficult to improve the geographical distribution of nurses in the United States.

The high turnover of hospital nurses, to summarize, is significant because it complicates the efforts of hospitals to maintain and increase effectiveness, reduces the productivity of the hospital by the costs it produces, makes hospitals reluctant to establish alternate career structures designed to improve nursing performance and patient care, and is one variable that contributes to the geographical maldistribution of hospital nurses in the United States. In short, the high rate of nursing turnover is significant because it has important consequences for the operation of American hospitals. And, to anticipate a later point, hospitals are a critically important part of the system of health-care delivery in the United States.

General Perspective[9]

Turnover is part of the general problem of organizational control. Organizations must produce an output to receive the resources necessary to operate. Hospitals, for instance, produce health-care services in return for money from their patients, insurance companies, and the government. All organizations, not just hospitals, must successfully solve the "economic problem" of resource acquisition. Production of an output, however, is not sufficient to maintain an effective organization. Organizations must also maintain members willing and able to perform the work necessary to produce the output which brings in the resources. Success at maintaining this performance, which is always prescribed by organizational norms, signifies solution of the "control problem" facing all organizations.

Turnover strikes at the foundation of organizational control. Norms specifying work to be done cannot be obeyed unless an organization can maintain its members. ("No members, no work," to adapt the traditional union slogan about work contracts into a new context.) And the greater the expenditure of scarce resources to maintain its membership, the more an organization must neglect the work necessary to produce its basic output. Organizations which neglect their basic output are likely to find their effectiveness drastically reduced. It is thus no wonder that high rates of turnover are of such concern to managers, since they recognize, better than most, the threat that these rates pose for the maintenance of effectiveness.

Problems of organizational control are manifested in behavior other than turnover. Absenteeism, strikes, employee theft, sickness and accidents (most of which are reflected in statistics about absenteeism), waste of materials, low levels of job performance (often termed "soldiering")—all represent behaviors which indicate, when the behaviors are excessive, than an organization is not successfully motivating its members to obey its official norms. Many of these behaviors are discussed under such social psychological labels are "morale" and "alienation." It is assumed, for instance, that employees with low morale will be absent more often than employees with high morale. Many of these behaviors are properly labeled as "deviant" because they represent significant departures from official organizational norms. Every instance of these behaviors, of course, does not result in reduced organizational effectiveness. As with turnover, some of these behaviors at times promote effectiveness. All of the behaviors, however, when excessive, signify serious problems of organizational control. What is important at this point is to relate turnover to these deviant behaviors and to view all of them in the general context of organizational control.

OUTLINE OF THE BOOK

This first chapter has defined the dependent variable of this research and indicated its significance. As previously indicated, the basis for the explanation of this turnover is a causal model developed from a review of the turnover literature. This model will be described in the second chapter. The data and methods used to estimate the model will be described in the third chapter. Results of the research will be presented in the fourth through the seventh chapters. Chapter 4 contains the results without controls, that is, the relationships between the determinants and turnover are examined without statistically removing the effects of the other variables in the causal model. The results with statistical controls are presented in Chapters 5 and 6. Chapter 5 contains the results for the entire sample of nurses, whereas Chapter 6 sets forth the findings for separate categories of nurses. Chapters 4, 5, and 6 use the nurse as the unit of analysis; Chapter 7, however, basically presents the findings, with and without statistical controls, for nursing units within the hospitals. The eighth and final chapter will mostly suggest ways to reduce the turnover of hospital nurses and will indicate how research on the determinants of turnover can be improved.

NOTES

1. The meaning of "crude turnover rate" is discussed in Price (1977, pp. 15-17).

2. The present situation could, of course, be different from the historical periods described in these studies. For some more recent data which suggest that the situation, at least with respect to nurses, has not basically changed, see Lysaught (1970, pp. 132, 146).

3. An extended discussion of the concept of turnover is found in Price (1977, pp. 4-9). Also helpful is Bluedorn (1978).

4. The following sources have been very helpful in providing background data for the material in this section: Altman (1972), Anderson (1968), Anderson (1978), Archibald (1971), Davis (1966), Lysaught (1970), Mauksch (1957, 1965), and Sloan (1975).

5. Propositions about organizational effectiveness are found in Price (1968); a discussion of the concept of effectiveness is contained in Price (1972b).

6. Two basic discussions of productivity are Fabricant (1969) and Kendrick (1977). Productivity is sometimes termed "efficiency" by sociologists.

7. See Price (1977, pp. 110-119) for an extended discussion of the impact of turnover on organizational effectiveness. Also helpful is the recent article by Dalton and Tudor (1979).

8. We recommend "alternate career structures" in Chapter 8 as a way to reduce the turnover of hospital nurses.

9. The discussion in this section is a simplified version of Talcott Parsons' material about "system problems." Johnson (1960, pp. 51-56) has a good summary of these systems problems.

CHAPTER 2
The Causal Model

Our objective in this chapter is to describe and discuss the causal model of turnover to be estimated in this study.[1] A causal model is a set of interrelated propositions. Each proposition states a relationship between an independent variable (commonly termed "X") and a dependent variable (commonly termed "Y"). We will follow the format whereby the propositions are stated as "successively higher amounts of X will likely produce successively higher amounts of Y." Although each proposition includes only two variables, the causal model, because it is a set of interrelated propositions, represents a multivariate system. In describing the expected interrelationships among these variables, we actually will be presenting a theory of turnover. We thus use the term "model" as equivalent to "theory."

A complete statement of a causal model requires specification of the linkages between the independent and dependent variables. Some of the linkages are explicit in the propositions. For example, in the preceding paragraph the illustrative proposition indicates a probabilistic relationship (the "likely" in the proposition) which is also positive. Although all of the propositions in our model are probabilistic rather than deterministic, some are negative rather than positive. Most of the linkages are not explicit in the propositions and must be specified in the discussion of the model. Our propositions are also linear rather than nonlinear, additive rather than multiplicative, and recursive rather than nonrecursive.

Both empirical and philosophical assumptions characterize causal models and should be specified to describe the model completely. An example of a basic philosophical assumption is that human behavior is orderly, whereas an example of an empirical assumption is that the independent variables are important to individuals.[2] Our concern will be only with the empirical assumptions.

The purpose of causal models is to provide an explanation of some phenomenon. Our model attempts to explain turnover and is based on the large body of literature on turnover.[3] As indicated in the preceding chapter, we will attempt to explain the turnover of hospital nurses. We wish to emphasize that use of the label "causal model" is not intended to convey a high level of theoretical and methodological sophistication. The model presented is intended to be a plausible summary of what is known about the determinants of turnover. Other causal arrangements of the variables are possible, perhaps even superior. In short, the model to be estimated is tentative and is very much a model in the process of being developed.

The model which we use to explain the turnover of hospital nurses is set forth in Table 2-1 and Figure 2-1. Table 2-1 contains verbal statements of the propositions in the model, whereas Figure 2-1 represents these propositions in diagrammatic form. Since turnover has already been defined and discussed, it remains to define and indicate theoretical and empirical support for variables in the model. All of these variables are referred to as "determinants" of turnover. However, as Figure 2-1 indicates, some of these determinants are intervening variables. Intent to stay, for example, intervenes between turnover and job satisfaction, professionalism, general training, and kinship responsibility. Job satisfaction intervenes between intent to stay, and routinization, participation, instrumental communication, integration, pay, distributive justice, and promotional opportunity. No variable intervenes between opportunity and turnover.

Table 2-1: The Causal Model of Turnover

Propositions
1. Successively higher amounts of intent to stay will likely produce successively lower amounts of turnover.
2. Successively higher amounts of job satisfaction will likely produce successively higher amounts of intent to stay.
3. Successively higher amounts of opportunity will likely produce successively higher amounts of turnover.
4. Successively higher amounts of routinization will likely produce successively lower amounts of job satisfaction.
5. Successively higher amounts of participation will likely produce successively higher amounts of job satisfaction.
6. Successively higher amounts of instrumental communication will likely produce successively higher amounts of job satisfaction.
7. Successively higher amounts of integration will likely produce successively higher amounts of job satisfaction.
8. Successively higher amounts of pay will likely produce successively higher amounts of job satisfaction.
9. Successively higher amounts of distributive justice will likely produce successively higher amounts of job satisfaction.
10. Successively higher amounts of promotional opportunity will likely produce successively higher amounts of job satisfaction.
11. Successively higher amounts of professionalism will likely produce successively lower amounts of intent to stay.
12. Successively higher amounts of general training will likely produce successively lower amounts of intent to stay.
13. Successively higher amounts of kinship responsibility will likely produce successively higher amounts of intent to stay.

THE CAUSAL MODEL

Intent to Stay

Intent to stay is the likelihood perceived by the individual of continued participation in the organization. Since intent to stay refers to individual perceptions rather than to individual behavior, it is a social psychological concept; it refers to the internal orientations of nurses and not to what they do. What we call intent to stay often is referred to as "commitment" and "identification" in the literature.

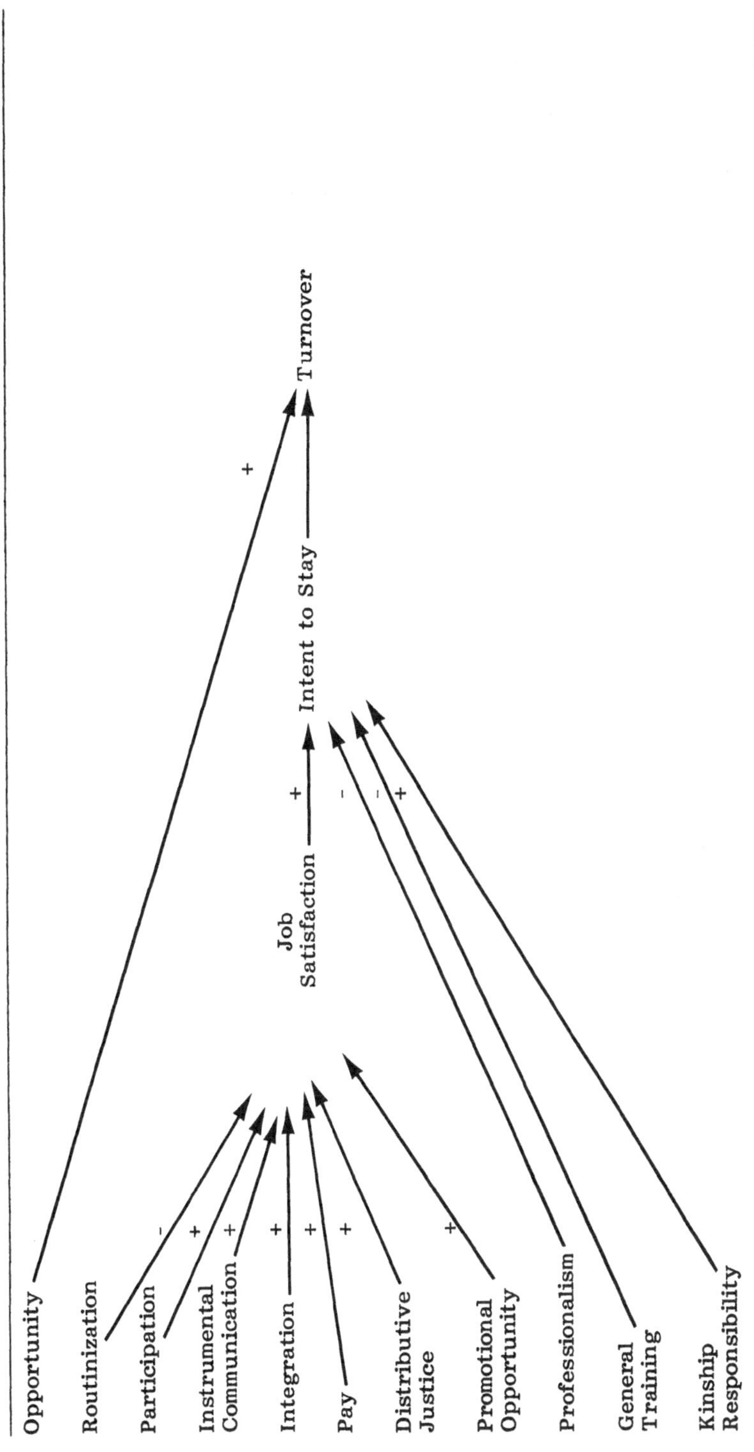

Figure 2-1: The Causal Model of Turnover

The important work of Porter and his colleagues on commitment is especially pertinent because they include intent to stay as one of their three dimensions of commitment.[4] "A strong belief in and acceptance of the organization's goals and values" and "a willingness to exert considerable effort on behalf of the organization" are their two other dimensions of commitment. The work of Porter and his colleagues is also important for our research because they have linked commitment to turnover.

There is a sizable body of literature (Atchinson and Lefferts 1972; Hunter 1962; Kraut 1975; Mangione 1973) which supports the idea that intent to stay has a negative impact on turnover, that is, the stronger the intent to stay, the less the likelihood of turnover. Mangione's research (1973) is illustrative. With information collected from 242 workers interviewed during a pretest for the 1969-1970 survey of working conditions, Mangione found (p. 343) that 75 percent of the workers who intended to stay with their present employers were still working with the same employers two years later. Fifty-nine percent of the workers who intended to leave actually left. Intent, whether to stay or leave, is related to subsequent behavior.

The literature about the more general concept of commitment can also be cited to support the intent-to-stay-turnover proposition. Mobley and his colleagues, in a careful review of the turnover literature which includes all the work by Porter and his colleagues, state (Mobley et al. 1979b, p. 508) that "the developing body of research on commitment" suggests that it is "significantly and negatively related to turnover."[5] Since intent to stay is but one dimension of commitment–at least in the Porter research–care must be exercised lest the impression be given that intent to stay equals commitment.

Job Satisfaction

Job satisfaction is the degree to which individuals like their work.[6] Nurses who indicate that they like their jobs are highly satisfied. The early literature dealing with this topic–the Western Electric research is a good example–commonly uses the term "morale," although more recent work, stimulated perhaps by the significant measurement work of Smith and her colleagues (1969), typically refers to this topic as "satisfaction." Satisfaction, like commitment, is a social psychological concept.

A large literature (Lawler 1973, pp. 62-63, 85, 101; Lefkowitz 1971; Lyons 1968, pp. 6-24; March and Simon 1958, p. 93; Pettman 1973; Porter and Steers 1973; Schuh 1967; Vroom 1964, pp. 175-187) supports the idea that increased job satisfaction directly reduces turnover. Vroom's widely cited review (1964) is illustrative of this literature. He states (p. 186) that "there is a consistent negative relationship between job satisfaction and the probability of resignation." "Resignation" in Vroom's review refers to voluntary separation from the organization. It should be emphasized that job satisfaction, in our view, is expected to increase the intent to stay, thus influencing turnover indirectly.

Some scholars question whether job satisfaction has an impact on turnover. In fact, many of the propositions of the causal model, with the possible exception of the opportunity-turnover proposition, are questioned by particular scholars, and these doubts are cited in the reviews which support the propositions. We do not claim total consensus for all the propositions in the model; we do claim, however, that all propositions in the model (with the exception of the Porter material about commitment) are supported by the bulk of the studies reviewed. Empirical research should, in the long run, resolve most of these questions.

There is little research which suggests, as we hypothesize in the model, that intent to stay is a variable which mediates the job-satisfaction-turnover relationship. The only example which could be located—and even here the relationships are not very explicit—is the sophisticated NORC study (1972) of the turnover of Roman Catholic priests. [7] The research on commitment, however, clearly views it as a variable that intervenes between job satisfaction and turnover. Mobley (1977), perhaps more than any other scholar, has explicitly indicated the mediating nature of commitment.[8] The job-satisfaction-and-commitment-turnover causal linkage is also implicit in the classic Porter and Steers review (1973) of the literature. In sum, despite the small amount of directly relevant data, the causal model presented here suggests that increased job satisfaction produces greater intent to stay, which, in turn, results in less turnover.

Finally, Porter and his colleagues are of the opinion, based on their research, that commitment is a more important determinant of turnover than job satisfaction. This is clearly a minority opinion among researchers in this area, since most of the literature on turnover does not even refer to commitment as a determinant, let alone assign it more importance than job satisfaction. A goal of our research is to assess the relative importance of intent to stay (a dimension of commitment) and job satisfaction as determinants of turnover.

Opportunity

Opportunity is the availability of alternative jobs in the organization's environment.[9] Economists commonly stress the importance of opportunity under diverse labels: "supply-demand," "pull," "level of employment," "economic conditions," "business cycles," and "state of the economy." Whereas commitment and job satisfaction refer to internal orientations of individuals, opportunity refers to a property of the organization's environment and is commonly measured by the number of job vacancies and the amount of unemployment: the greater the number of job vacancies, the greater the opportunity, and the greater the amount of unemployment, the less the opportunity.

Opportunity's positive impact on turnover is supported by a substantial body of literature (Bowey 1974, p. 16; Burton and Parker 1969; Fry 1973; March and Simon 1958, p. 101; Pettman 1973). The review by March and Simon (1958), probably the most influential statement about the determinants of turnover, well illustrates this. They state (p. 101) that "when jobs are plentiful, voluntary movement is high; when jobs are scarce, voluntary turnover is small." Transposed into the terms of our research, March and Simon are asserting that increases in opportunity produce increases in turnover.

Intervening variables are not commonly suggested; instead, increased opportunity is assumed to increase directly the amount of turnover.[10] Recent work by Bluedorn (1976) and Martin (1977), however, suggests job satisfaction as an intervening variable between opportunity and turnover. The Bluedorn and Martin research is another minority position which will be examined in our research.

There currently exists no way whereby the various determinants can be ranked in terms of their relative impact on turnover. Such ranking is impossible because no research has included all the suggested determinants in the same model—thus allowing for the simultaneous control of other determinants while examining the influence of any particular one. March and Simon (1958) comment on ranking in their discussion of the determinants of turnover; they believe (p. 101), in the absence of systematic empirical evidence, that opportunity is the most important determinant of turnover. An important goal of our research is to indicate the relative influence of all the major determinants in terms of their impact on turnover. We will thus be able to assess empirically March and Simon's claim.

The literature supporting the positive impact of opportunity on turnover makes two assumptions. First, it is assumed that the members of the organization have knowledge about the alternative jobs in the environment. There is some literature supporting this assumption. Mattila, for instance, notes (1974, p. 235) that "at least 50 to 60 percent of all workers line up their new jobs before quitting and leaving their old jobs." Workers who "line up their new jobs" have knowledge about the opportunity available to them, and "quitting" is, of course, synonymous with voluntary separation. Second, it is assumed that members of the organization have the freedom to enter and leave the organization. Restrictions on this freedom are typically imposed by the state, as when in June, 1940 all the workers in the Soviet Union were frozen in their jobs (Fainsod 1963, p. 107). Since this freedom characterizes all contemporary Western societies, this second assumption is empirically sound for the research reported here.

Intent to stay and job satisfaction are, as previously indicated, social psychological concepts; they refer to internal orientations of individuals. Opportunity, on the other hand, refers to an objective characteristic of the organization's environment, the number of alternative jobs available in the labor market. The next seven determinants of turnover, like opportunity, do not refer to internal orientations. Like intent to stay and job satisfaction, however, the next seven determinants do refer to individual properties.

Routinization

Routinization is the degree to which a job is repetitive, with high routinization signifying a high degree of repetitiveness.[11] Routinization is commonly treated in the organizational literature in discussions of "technology," where, as a rule, it is one form of technology. "Variety" is another commonly used term which has the same referent as routinization, except that high variety indicates low routinization.

A smaller body of literature (Argyris 1960, p. 14; Baldamus 1951; Goodman et al. 1973; Lawler 1973, pp. 159-163; Porter and Steers 1973) consistently indicates that increases in routinization produce increases in turnover. The classic Porter and Steers review (1973) is illustrative of this literature. They note (p. 164) that "the available data tend to indicate" that turnover is "positively associated with task repetitiveness." "Task repetitiveness" corresponds to our "routinization." Porter and Steers also indicate that the routinization-turnover proposition must be viewed as tentative.

The literature which supports the routinization-turnover proposition implicitly treats job satisfaction as an intervening variable. Increases in routinization decrease job satisfaction, which, in turn, increases turnover. The Porter and Steers review is also an example of the implicit use of job satisfaction as an intervening variable. They note (p. 162) that increases in routinization, in the language of our research, results in greater "job stress," which, in turn, increases turnover. The context of "job stress" indicates that it is the converse of our "job satisfaction."

Job satisfaction as an intervening variable is also implicit in the literature supporting the next six determinants of turnover. In the interest of economy, however, citations which provide such implicit causal ordering will not be included.

Participation

Participation is the degree of power an individual exercises concerning performance of the job. Literature about participation is commonly found in discussions of "centralization" and "autonomy."[12] When hospitals, for instance, are highly centralized, nurses have a low degree of participation, and when nurses exercise a high degree of autonomy, their participation is high. Centralization and autonomy are, respectively, organizational and individual properties. Participation is, of course, also an individual property. It is important to note that participation does not refer to power relating to major (and many minor) organizational decisions, but is limited to power to influence the immediate job.[13]

Numerous studies (Argyris 1973; Farris 1971; Goodman et al. 1973; Knowles 1964; Lawler 1973 pp. 152-153, 158-159, 163, 190; Lefkowitz 1971; March and Simon 1958, p. 95; Pettman 1973; Porter and Steers 1973) indicate that high participation results in low turnover. For example, Pettman, working in the March and Simon tradition, notes (pp. 48-49) "that the greater the individual's participation in job assignment," the "lower the turnover rate." "Participation in job assignment" is one form of power concerning the job. Our causal model, however, portrays participation as having its influence on turnover indirectly through job satisfaction, which, in turn, influences intent to stay.

Instrumental Communication

Instrumental communication is the degree to which information about the job is transmitted by an organization to its members (Price 1977, pp. 58-59). When instrumental communication is high, individuals are well informed about their jobs. Material pertinent to instrumental communication is often found in discussions of "role clarity" and "feedback." A high amount of instrumental communication typically means that role clarity and feedback are high. Employees who are given "realistic job previews" are also characterized by high amounts of instrumental communication. Instrumental communication refers to a behavioral property of an individual's job, that is, how well the individual is informed about work by the organization. As with participation, the limited focus of instrumental communication should be emphasized; the concept does not refer to the transmission of gossip or strategic organizational plans, but is limited to job-related information.

As with participation, there is considerable literature (Lawler 1973; pp. 160-163; Levine and Wright 1957; Scott 1972; Wanous 1973; Wieland 1969) supporting a negative impact of instrumental communication on turnover. The influential work of Lawler (1973) is a good example of this literature. He notes (pp. 160-163) that high "feedback about what is accomplished" satisfies employees and produces low turnover.[14] Feedback about job accomplishments is, of course, one type of instrumental communication. More than most authors, Lawler explicitly locates job satisfaction as a variable that intervenes between instrumental communication and turnover.[15] Our model shows increased instrumental communication resulting in higher job satisfaction, which increases intent to stay, which, in turn, decreases the probability of turnover.

Integration

Integration is the degree to which an individual has close friends among organizational members.[16] Many close friends signifies high integration. Most of these close friends, in contemporary Western organizations, will not generally be members of the same kinship network. In fact, organizations commonly prefer not to have relatives working together. The organizational literature dealing with "primary groups" is relevant and indicates that where there is a high degree of participation in primary groups, integration is high. It should be emphasized that integration is a characteristic of the individual (the number of close friends at work) that is visible to an outside observer and does not refer to an internal orientation.

There is strong support in the literature (Knowles 1964; Lawler 1973; pp. 17, 195; Lefkowitz 1971; Pettman 1973; Porter and Steers 1973; Schuh 1967; Van der Merwe and Miller 1971, 1973) for a negative impact of integration on turnover. Van der Merwe and Miller (1971, 1973) have strongly emphasized the significance of integration in their important work on turnover. They note (1971, p. 239), for example, that "a major need satisfier is likely to be that of belonging to a cohesive and rewarding group, and if this need is not satisfied, the worker will very likely fail to adjust to the work situation and will therefore more readily withdraw from it." A "cohesive and rewarding group" is likely to be one which is high on integration, and workers who "withdraw" from a group, in Van der Merwe and Miller's research, are examples of turnover. Our model indicates that integration influences turnover indirectly through job satisifaction and intent to stay.

The basis for including integration in most contemporary research on turnover, though this particular label is not used, is the Western Electric research. Of especial importance in this connection is Mayo and Lombard's World War II study (1944) of the aircraft industry of southern California.[17] In Great Britain, the significant work of the Tavistock Institute of Human Relations on turnover is also in the Western Electric research tradition, as is the work of Van der Merwe and Miller.[18]

The previous discussion of opportunity indicated that the relative importance of the determinants of turnover cannot be specified because all of the major determinants have not been included in the same model. March and Simon, it may be recalled, argue (1958, p. 101) that opportunity is the most important determinant of turnover. Van der Merwe and Miller, however, designate (1970, p. 24) integration, as defined here, as the major determinant of turnover. A major goal of our research is to arrive at a ranking of these determinants so that debates such as these can be settled.

Pay

Pay refers to money and its equivalents, such as fringe benefits, which individuals receive for their services to the organization (Lawler 1971, p. 1). Since the equivalents of money are very difficult to measure, most research on pay uses direct cash income as the measure of pay. It should be emphasized that "pay" refers not to "satisfaction with pay" (a social psychological variable) but to the amount of direct cash income received by individuals (a variable which could be obtained from organizational records).

The literature (Dowey 1974, pp. 15-16; Burton and Parker 1969; Fry 1973; Goodman et al. 1973; Lawler 1973, pp. 95-96; Pencavel 1970, pp. 10-19; Porter and Steers 1973; Stoikov and Raimon 1968) strongly supports a negative relationship between pay and turnover: increases in pay produce decreases in turnover. Pencavel, for instance, notes (p. 22) that "the depressing effect of the level of wages on quits seems well established."[19] "Wages" and "quits," of course, correspond respectively to our "pay" and "turnover." Our model states that pay influences turnover indirectly through job satisfaction and intent to stay.

There are data which place in doubt the negative relationship between pay and turnover. Some of these data, when examined carefully, turn out not to contradict the suggested proposition, but to qualify it in various ways. However, for pay, as for some of the other determinants, some contradictory data always remain. This is to be expected in scientific research. All that is claimed for the propositions of the causal model is that they summarize the main thrust of the literature on turnover. In time, the contradictory data will have to be reconciled with the bulk of the literature. But for the present, our contention is that the propositions are consistent with most of the literature.[20]

Many scholars, especially economists, assign primary importance to pay as a determinant of turnover, and there is probably more literature supporting pay than any other determinant, with the possible exception of opportunity. It is possible that pay has received so much attention because it is relatively easy to measure. (Ease of measurement may also account for some of the importance assigned to opportunity.) However, as indicated in the discussions on opportunity and integration, the relative importance of these variables can be assessed only when all the possible determinants are in the same model.

A considerable segment of the literature, especially that produced by social psychologists, emphasizes the importance of individual variation concerning the determinants of turnover.[21] This emphasis is especially prominent in discussions of pay where the point is made that pay will be a significant determinant of turnover only if it is highly valued; when it is not highly valued, it will cease to have an important impact on turnover.[22] The emphasis on individual variations is sound; such differences do exist. However, there are also norms which prescribe what the individual should desire, and these norms are commonly supported by the individual's experience. In particular, success is often measured by pay, and work organizations reinforce this standard for evaluation with their reward structure. In our research, it is assumed that all of the determinants are of sufficient importance to motivate the behavior of the individuals studied.[23]

Distributive Justice

Distributive justice is the degree to which rewards and punishments are related to performance inputs into the organization (Homans 1961, pp. 232-264). When distributive justice is high in the nursing department of a hospital, for instance, the nurses who work hard receive more rewards (pay, recognition, and power), whereas the nurses who only "put in their time" receive fewer rewards and are, in effect, punished. Hard work is but one type of performance input into the organization; increased education and experience are examples of other inputs. Material relevant to distributive justice is found in discussions of such social psychological concepts as equity and fairness. When rewards and punishments of nurses, to return to our previous example, are related to their performance inputs, it is likely that the nurses will perceive their situation to be equitable or fair. Distributive justice refers not to the amounts of rewards and punishments distributed, but to the relationship between rewards-punishments and performance inputs. It is this relationship rather than the amount which is critical in defining distributive justice.

There is a modest amount of literature (Carrell and Dittrich 1978; Cole 1971, pp. 72-132; Goodman et al. 1973; Gowler 1969; Lawler 1973, p. 144; Porter and Steers 1973; Telly et al. 1971; Valenzi and Andrews 1971) which indicates that distributive justice reduces turnover. The review of the literature of the hard-core unemployed by Goodman et al., for instance, notes (p. 27) that "the fairness of treatment by the counselor during training is positively related to job retention." "Fairness of treatment" illustrates one dimension of distributive justice and "job retention" indicates a lack of turnover. Our model depicts increased distributive justice as producing greater job satisfaction, which, in turn, reduces turnover by increasing intent to stay.

Although there is a modest amount of literature which supports the distributive-justice-turnover proposition, it is possible that its significance is underestimated by the literature. Much of the research pertinent to distributive justice has been performed in laboratory experiments by social psychologists, and these experiments do not generally deal with turnover. When distributive justice is related to turnover outside of laboratory experiments, it is not part of a model which includes all the major determinants of turnover. Hence, judgement about the relative importance of distributive justice awaits the type of test provided by our research.

Promotional Opportunity

Promotional opportunity is the degree of potential vertical occupational mobility within an organization (Price 1977, p. 88). Promotional opportunity will, for instance, be high when a hospital is highly complex (many units and a long chain of command) and when promotions are exclusively from within the hospital.[24] Material relevant to promotional opportunity is often contained in discussions of "blocked mobility." Although it is commonly measured perceptually, as are the other behavioral determinants of this research, promotional opportunity is intended to be an objective variable because it refers to the actual possibility for an individual to get ahead in an organization.

There are some data which indicate that promotional opportunity is negatively related to turnover, that is, the more the promotional opportunity, the less the turnover (Cole 1971, pp. 101-135; Herzberg et al. 1957, p. 62; Ladinsky 1967; Lawler 1973, p. 131; Porter and Steers 1973). Porter and Steers, for instance, observe (p. 186) that "promotional considerations often appear to represent significant factors in the termination decision." In the language of our research, low promotional opportunity produces turnover. There are many studies which indicate the importance of promotional opportunity for job satisfaction. Much of this literature, however, does not deal with turnover and cannot be cited to support the causal model.

The preceding seven determinants (routinization, participation, instrumental communication, integration, pay, distributive justice, and promotional opportunity) are believed to have an impact on turnover through job satisfaction and intent to stay. The latter two concepts are the intervening variables through which the seven determinants influence turnover. Job satisfaction, as previously indicated, is mostly implicitly assumed by other researchers to intervene between these seven determinants and turnover. And only recently, as was discussed, has it been explicitly suggested that intent to stay (as a dimension of commitment)might serve as an intervening variable between job satisfaction and turnover. Intent to stay might, of course, serve as an intervening variable between some of these seven determinants and turnover without job satisfaction being involved. Salancik's (1977) stimulating review of the commitment literature suggests this possibility for instrumental communications, centralization and, perhaps, integration. These possibilities, although not incorporated formally into the causal model because of the lack of empirical support, will be checked in our research. The model also indicates, to emphasize an earlier observation, that opportunity is believed to have a direct impact on turnover; the literature on opportunity seldom mentions job satisfaction and commitment as intervening variables in the opportunity-turnover proposition.

The remaining three determinants appear to influence turnover only indirectly through intent to stay. Whereas it was easy to document the intervening nature of job satisfaction for the preceding seven determinants—although this was not always done, in the interest of economy—it is more difficult to document the intervening nature of intent to stay for the remaining three determinants. In addition, it is possible that these remaining three determinants have an impact on job satisfaction as well as on intent to stay. No literature could be located to support these relationships. Our analysis strategy, however, will allow us to check these possibilities.

Professionalism

Professionalism is the degree of dedication by individuals to occupational standards of performance; the greater the dedication to occupational standards, the greater the professionalism.[25] As a rule, professionalism appears to vary with the extent to which an occupation is based on systematized and generalized knowledge. Medicine, for example, has more knowledge of this type than nursing, and physicians generally appear to be characterized by greater professionalism than nurses. Literature relevant to professionalism is often found in discussions of "cosmopolitans" and "locals," where cosmopolitans are typically defined as having a higher degree of professionalism than locals. The term "dedication" in the definition is intended to have a behavioral referent. Nurses characterized by a high degree of professionalism, for example, exhibit, by their behavior, greater adherence to the performance standards emphasized by the nursing profession than nurses characterized by a low degree of professionalism.

It is generally believed, though without too much empirical support, that increased professionalism results in greater turnover (Blau 1973, p. 197; Caplow and McGee 1958; Carlson 1962, pp. 61-68; Charters 1954; Corwin 1961; Flango and Brumbaugh 1974; Gouldner 1957, 1958; Grusky 1964, p. 85; Kramer 1968, 1974, pp. 67-103; Kramer and Baker 1971). Flango and Brumbaugh's study (1974) of university faculty members in Pennsylvania illustrates this proposition. They find (p. 202) that cosmopolitans "were more likely to leave the institution with which they were presently affiliated" than were locals. One difference between the cosmopolitans and locals is greater "commitment to professional skills" by the cosmopolitans. Commitment to professional skills is a close approximation to our dedication to occupational standards of performance. In short, the cosmopolitans exhibited more professionalism than the locals. Cosmopolitans and locals who leave universities in Pennsylvania are, of course, exhibiting turnover.

The means whereby increased professionalism produces greater turnover is not too clear. The research on cosmopolitans and locals typically–and here Gouldner's seminal research (1957, 1958) on a small private liberal arts college is especially relevant–locates (1957, p. 290) the cosmopolitans' greater turnover in less "loyalty to the employing organization," greater "commitment to professional skills," and more frequent external "reference group orientations." It appears to us that a high degree of professionalism ("commitment to professional skills") results in strong orientations to the profession rather than to the employing organization (external "reference group orientations"), which, in turn, lead to less intent to stay in the employing organization ("loyalty to the employing organization"), which, finally, produces greater turnover. In brief, we view intent to stay as a variable that intervenes between professionalism and turnover. Our view seems to be a reasonable interpretation of some of the key studies of cosmopolitans and locals, and one purpose of our research is to subject this interpretation to a systematic empirical test.

Most of the research to support the professionalism-turnover proposition, like that of Flango and Brumbaugh (1974) and Gouldner (1957, 1958), cited above, is conducted on college professors. After college professors, research scientists are perhaps the next most frequently studied occupation. There is thus some question as to whether this proposition is applicable to hospital nurses.[26] Kramer (1968, 1974, pp. 67-103; Kramer and

Baker 1971), however, has studied turnover among hospital nurses, and her important research is consistent with the professionalism-turnover proposition.[27]

General Training

General training is the degree to which the occupational socialization of an individual results in the ability to increase the productivity of diverse organizations.[28] The training of a physician, for instance, is very general because it provides the ability to work effectively in most types of hospitals. On the other hand, the training of a specialist on military weapons in the U.S. Air Force, such as an operator of a cruise missile, is very specific because it provides the ability to work in no organizations outside the United States military command. The emphasis on general training comes from the literature on human capital in economics where it is noted that ability is a form of human capital and is a means whereby organizational productivity is increased. Amount of formal schooling is often used as a measure of general training: the greater the formal schooling, the greater the general training. In contrast, "on-the-job" training is typically very organization-specific. "Training," it should be noted, is not intended to be a derogatory term, as in the "training of an animal," but instead is intended to be broad enough to include occupational socialization in a university and on-the-job instruction by one's peers.

There is a small amount of data which support the proposition that increased general training results in greater turnover. Becker suggests (1964, p. 24) such a relationship in his seminal work on human capital when he states that "turnover should be least for employees with extremely specific training and most for those receiving...general training." Becker, however, provides no empirical data to support the suggested general-training-turnover proposition. Some empirical data to support the proposition are provided by Parsons (1972) in his study of layoffs and quits in American manufacturing industries.[29] He finds (p. 1140) "strong support" for the idea "that average quit and layoff rates" are lower in "industries where worker- and firm-financed specific investments are heavy." Where "specific investments are heavy," general training is low and turnover is correspondingly reduced. As previously indicated, we are concerned with quits and not layoffs.

Since there are few data supporting the suggested positive impact of general training on turnover, there has been almost no concern with how such a relationship comes about. In short, the intervening variable(s) has not been specified. Such lack of specification is understandable because the economists who have proposed the proposition almost exclusively use secondary data provided by the federal government of the United States. Parsons, for instance, uses data from the Bureau of Labor Statistics and the Census Bureau. Secondary data of this type seldom provide sufficient information to estimate intervening variables.

We are of the opinion that general training influences turnover through intent to stay. Individuals with general training would seem to have less intention to stay with the employer than individuals with specific training. This influence of intent to stay would primarily be the result of the location of the training. General training takes place outside the premises of the employer, whereas specific training is provided on the job. In our research, baccalaureate nurses have more general training than diploma nurses because the former are trained in universities and colleges, while the latter are trained in hospitals. It is, of course, possible that the impact of general training on turnover could also be mediated by job satisfaction, and this possibility will be assessed in our research.

Kinship Responsibility

Kinship responsibility is the degree of an individual's obligations to relatives in the community in which the employer is located.[30] Marriage, children, and relatives are the sources of increased kinship responsibility, and the greater the number of local kin, the greater the kinship responsibility. The idea of kinship responsibility corresponds approximately to the idea of "family responsibility" used in some of the turnover literature (Porter and Steers 1973).[31]

Kinship responsibility as a possible determinant of turnover was suggested to us by the literature on migration in demography (Comay 1972; Leslie and Richardson 1961; Long 1972; Miller 1976). Long, for instance, using data from the Current Population Survey, states (1972, p. 382) that "ages of children emerge as a major source of migration differentials." Implicit in Long's research is the idea that parental responsibility varies with the ages of children. And parental responsibility is, of course, one type of kinship responsibility. Much migration probably does not involve turnover. Executives, for instance, who are transferred from one part of the country to another are counted as migrants but not quits. However, some turnover is included in the migration statistics, and it seems plausible to us that the determinants of migration might also be determinants of turnover.

The migration literature does not indicate how kinship responsibility, to use the terms of our research, produces variations in turnover. We suggest that increased kinship responsibility reduces turnover by increasing the nurse's intent to stay. It is easiest to fulfill kinship obligations by continued residence in the community. Obligations are also fulfilled with greater ease by continued work with the same employer. Since the employer is located in the same community as the kinship members, continued employment with the same employer is, in effect, a means to comply with kinship obligations with the least possible burden–the result should be increased intent to stay with the employer.

Discussions of the determinants of turnover also refer to variables which this research labels "correlates," often called "demographic variables" by other researchers. If the causal model is to be a plausible summary of the literature concerning the determinants of turnover, the place of the correlates in the model must be indicated, and it is to this topic that we now turn.

CORRELATES

Age and length of service are probably the most commonly cited correlates in the literature. Level of skill, occupation, and education are also widely cited. As is suggested by these examples, most of the commonly used correlates refer to the properties of individuals. Some correlates refer to the properties of organizations, however–examples are the existence of a union and whether or not investments in the pension fund are transferable when an individual leaves the organization. Still other correlates refer to the properties of countries, such as the employment rate. Therefore, it is important to remember that the units of analysis for correlates vary.

The correlates are not included in the causal model because they do not indicate the means whereby they produce variations in turnover. Age may be used to illustrate this point. There is substantial literature (Price 1977, pp. 28-29) which supports a negative relationship between age and turnover: younger members of an organization usually have higher rates of turnover than older members. Age refers to span of years lived and is usually measured by asking respondents, either verbally or by questionnaire, to indicate how old they are. However, span of years lived does not indicate what is is about these years that has a negative impact on turnover. Older organizational members differ in significant ways from younger members, and the exact content of these differences must be explicitly stated. The content of these differences is explicitly stated in the variables in Table 2-1 and Figure 2-1. Younger members, for instance, usually have higher rates of turnover than older members because they – the younger members – usually have the most routine jobs, participate little in decision making, lack knowledge about their jobs, have fewer close friends, receive less pay, and have few local obligations to kin. In sum, it is not age itself that produces variations in turnover, but the variables commonly associated with age, that is, routinization, centralization, instrumental communications, integration, pay, and kinship responsibility.[32]

The correlates of turnover will not be totally ignored, however. When the procedures are discussed in the next chapter, two important uses of the correlates will be discussed.

INNOVATIVENESS OF THE CAUSAL MODEL

The major innovative feature claimed for the causal model is its comprehensiveness.[33] This feature of the model is exhibited in two ways. First, much research on the determinants of turnover commonly ignores important variables. Economists, for example, typically focus on pay and opportunity to the exclusion of other determinants. Noneconomists, typically social psychologists and sociologists, often focus on routinization, centralization, and so forth, and ignore pay and opportunity. Our model includes variables stressed by both economists and noneconomists. Second, much research on the sources of turnover does not specify the means whereby a determinant is believed to produce variations in turnover. In short, the intervening variables are not explicitly indicated. The best example of this lack of specification is for the correlates of turnover, as described in the preceding section. This lack of specification is also abundantly illustrated in the common failure to indicate explicitly the intervening nature of job satisfaction and intent to stay.[34]

This greater comprehensiveness of the model should allow for better explanation of turnover and provide the basis for ordering the determinants. As a rule, the explanatory power of a model increases as the number of variables included in the model increases. And the model described in this chapter has more determinants than other models. Since most research has not tested comprehensive models of turnover, it has not been possible to order the determinants by their explanatory power. The amount of supporting data, as was repeatedly noted in the preceding discussion of the model, does not provide an adequate base for ranking the determinants. This research, since it estimates a comprehensive model, should provide a means to order the determinants.

NOTES

1. The discussion of causal model in this section is much indebted to the work of Zetterberg (1965). The term "causal model," however, is not used by Zetterberg, who prefers the label "theory." The following sources have also been very helpful in thinking about causal models: Homans (1967), Merton (1957, pp. 85-101), Parsons (1949, pp. 3-42), Duncan (1966), Land (1969), Heise (1969), and Jöreskog and Sorböm (1978).

2. Pay, for example, is posited as an important determinant of turnover. If pay does have this impact on turnover, it means that pay is im-

portant to individuals in the organization. If pay is not important it will not serve to motivate behavior. This is an assumption which is capable of being empirically checked. Material will be presented about this and other assumptions throughout the chapter.

3. Detailed documentation for our causal model is contained in Price (1977, pp. 66-91). We have attempted in this chapter to present mostly the major sources supporting our model. Strongly supported determinants, in some instances, seem to be based on less data than weakly supported determinants. This apparent difference is the result of the fact that the sources cited differ in extensiveness. Some of the sources review large amounts of literature, whereas other sources refer only to single empirical studies. The amount of supporting data is not indicated by the number of citations.

4. An excellent review of the work of Porter and his colleagues on commitment is contained in Mowday et al. (1979). Their definition of commitment is found on pp. 225-226.

5. Also relevant is Mobley (1977) and Mobley et al. (1978, 1979a). Earlier work on commitment was performed by Marsh and Mannari (1971, 1972). We focus mostly on the work of Porter and his colleagues because of the dominant position which their work now occupies in the research on commitment.

6. Some version of this definition is used in much of the literature dealing with job satisfaction. The terms may change but the idea is widespread in the literature.

7. Also relevant is Greeley (1972) and Schoenherr and Greeley (1974).

8. Brief and Aldag's work (1977) is also pertinent here.

9. This definition is implicit in the measures of many of the economists who do research on turnover. They often operationally rather than nominally define opportunity.

10. Price (1977, pp. 81-83) has suggested that opportunity be treated as an intervening variable. This is a plausible position. However, most of the literature suggests that opportunity has a direct impact on turnover, and it is this latter position which we now adopt.

11. This concept is suggested by the work of Perrow (1967).

12. Literature about participation is also found in discussions of alienation. Our measurement of participation corresponds to the most widely used definition of alienation, powerlessness. See Kanungo (1979) for an excellent discussion of the literature about alienation.

13. A discussion of power is found in Price (1972a, p. 36).

14. Lawler also notes (1973, pp. 160-163) that high feedback produces low absenteeism and high quality of work performed.

15. Motivation, according to Lawler (1973, pp. 160-163), also intervenes between instrumental communication and turnover.

16. This definition of integration was stimulated by Blau's work (1959-60, 1960a) using this term. Blau, however, does not define integration as we do.

17. Also relevant is Mayo (1924).

18. There is a sizable amount of literature on turnover published by researchers at the Tavistock Institute. Good introductions to a major portion of this literature are provided by Hill (1952) and Rice (1953).

19. Also relevant is Pencavel (1972).

20. The only exception to this, to emphasize a previous note, is our treatment of job satisfaction, commitment, and turnover. Most of the literature on turnover does not, as we do, view commitment as an intervening variable between job satisfaction and turnover. As indicated earlier in this chapter, we adopt what appears to be the more plausible, but deviant, position of Porter and his colleagues (Mowday et al. 1979).

21. The work of Lawler (1971, 1973) is often cited in these discussions of individual variation. Much of the emphasis on individual variation is, however, the result of Vroom's (1964) major book on work and motivation.

22. Ingham's work (1967, 1970) is often used to document the significance of individual variation concerning the importance of pay.

23. Since it is so widely discussed in the literature, we did check for interaction effects between pay and the importance of pay. No interaction effects were found.

24. Complexity is discussed in Price (1972a, pp. 70-71).

25. When professionalism is viewed from an individual perspective rather than from an occupational viewpoint (and our research adopts an individual perspective), it seems to us that the core of its meaning centers on the degree of dedication to occupational standards of performance. Although we do not adopt their definitions, since they view professionalism from an occupational perspective, we have been very much helped in thinking about these matters by the classic work of Goode (1960), Friedson (1971), and Wilensky (1964).

26. This question may, of course, be raised about all of our propositions. The question, however, seems to be especially appropriate here since most of the research on professionalism has been devoted to occupations very different from hospital nursing.

27. Also relevant is Brief (1976).

28. This definition is based on the work of Becker (1962; 1964, p. 18).

29. Also relevant is Parsons (1973).

30. As far as we are aware, this is our idea. The idea occurred to us while reviewing the demographic literature on migration.

31. Note also the work of Tainio (1977, pp. 37-38).

32. Evidence for some of these associations is found in the following sources: Beattie and Spencer (1971), Peterson and Schoenherr (1978), Stolzenberg (1975), and Wright and Hamilton (1978). Most of our "evidence" for these associations, however, comes from our general impressions about the manner in which organizations operate.

33. The most important excluded determinant is size. The nature of the relationship between size and turnover is ambiguous (Price 1977, pp. 89-90). We could not estimate the model for size since all of our hospitals are essentially the same size, as will be indicated in the following chapter. We did, however, estimate the model for size of the nursing units; the data for this estimation are in Appendix 7-1. Most of the literature about size refers to the organization (the hospital) rather than to the subjects within the organizations (the nursing units). There is also some evidence supporting coordination and effectiveness as determinants; the data indicate that increased coordination (Lyons 1968) and increased effectiveness (Eitzen and Yetman 1972; Grusky 1960; Hirschman 1970, p. 102; Pfeffer and Salancik 1978, p. 238) produce a reduction in turnover. We did not include coordination and effectiveness in our causal model because they have a very restricted data base. Only one study supports coordination, and most of the evidence for effectiveness comes from research on executive succession, which is only marginally relevant for turnover. Coordination and effectiveness were also included in Price's pilot study (Price and Bluedorn 1979), where they were not important determinants of turnover. Price's pilot study also suggested the possibility that increased community participation, viewed as involvement in voluntary associations, might reduce turnover. Community participation was of some importance in the pilot study, but when estimated in the present study it had no net impact on turnover. To simplify the discussion of the model, we have omitted any consideration of community participation. For some information about psychological determinants, see Price (1977, p. 137).

34. Some of the research on the impact of job satisfaction on turnover also does not indicate the determinants of job satisfaction. Specification of these determinants is, of course, an important feature of our causal model.

CHAPTER 3
Data and Methods

This chapter describes the data and methods used to estimate the causal model set forth in the preceding chapter. Five topics will be treated: site, sample, data collection, measurement, and data analysis.

SITE

The site of this research is seven voluntary, short-term general hospitals. Basic information about the hospitals is contained in Table 3-1. Four characteristics of the hospitals are noteworthy. (1) Six of the hospitals are of medium size, that is, their bed capacity is between 100 and 500. Even the seventh hospital, with 620 beds, is basically a medium-sized hospital.[1] (2) All of the hospitals are located in the north central part of the United States (Wattenberg and Scammon 1965, p. 332), and are, in popular terminology, part of the "Midwest." (3) The communities in which the hospitals are located are also of medium size, with populations between 50,000 and 250,000 (U.S. Bureau of the Census 1970, C15, p. 326, and C17, p. 209). Almost 15 percent of the American population lives is communities of this size (U.S. Bureau of the Census 1975, p. 19). (4) All of the hospitals are church-operated; four are Protestant and three are Roman Catholic.

Since a random sample of hospitals was not studied, the universe to which the results of our research can be generalized is not clear. The results should, of course, be most applicable to hospitals similar to those studied. It is our hope, however, that the results will be applicable considerably beyond the types of hospitals studied, but only time and further research will indicate the extent to which the results can be generalized.

To elaborate on our discussion in Chapter 1, hospitals were selected as a site for two reasons. First, they are a major source of direct health care in the United States. Most members of the health occupations are, for example, employed by hospitals (U.S. National Center for Health Statistics 1976, p. 25). In 1976, 60 percent of the physicians, dentists, nurses, technologists, dieticians, therapists, and health-service workers were hospital employees. Although physicians are seldom hospital employees-only about 26 percent of all physicians and dentists are employed by hospitals–they typically treat their more serious cases of illness in hospitals, and are thus very dependent on the facilities of the hospitals.[2]

Table 3-1: Characteristics of the Hospitals Studied

Hospital	Number of Beds [a]	State	Size of Community [b]	Church Affiliation [a]
1	350	Illinois	217,380	Protestant
2	281	Illinois	217,380	Protestant
3	276	Iowa	217,380	Protestant
4	406	Iowa	110,642	Catholic
5	390	Iowa	62,314	Catholic
6	620	Iowa	110,642	Protestant
7	280	Iowa	217,380	Catholic

a American Hospital Association, Hospitals: Guide Issue, 1976, pp. 66-75 and 79-84.

b U.S. Bureau of the Census, Census of Population: 1970, General Social and Economic Characteristics, Final Report, PC(1)-C15 and C17, Illinois and Iowa, p. 326 and p. 209.

The second reason for studying hospitals is that they are a service organization. Most of the research on turnover has been conducted on organizations that provide goods rather than services, especially manufacturing organizations (Organization for Economic Cooperation and Development 1965, p. 110). The emphasis on organizations that provide goods is to be expected since such organizations have been the dominant type of organization in the United States. Only recently have service organizations become of major importance (Bell 1973; Fuchs 1968). Since the causal model described in the preceding chapter is based mostly on the study of goods-producing organizations, there is the reasonable question of its applicability to service-producing organizations. Our research will assess the extent to which the model is appropriate to one type of service organization, hospitals.[3]

Voluntary, short-term general hospitals were selected because they are the most common type of hospital in the United States (American Hospital Association 1977, pp. 66-75, 79-84). In 1976, there were approximately 7,082 hospitals in the United States. Of these, 3,368, or about 48 percent, were voluntary, short-term general hospitals. The next largest category is the 1,836 (about 26 percent) state and local hospitals. Since hospitals are a major organization in the provision of direct health-care delivery in the United States, and since voluntary, short-term general hospitals are the dominant type of hospital in the United States, our research focuses on a critical segment of the health-care-delivery system in the United States.

SAMPLE

The sample consists of the nonsupervisory registered nurses. Supervisory nurses were excluded to simplify the analysis. Model estimation is easiest with homogeneous samples since possible confounding variables are eliminated by selection. Since supervisory personnel generally have lower rates of turnover than nonsupervisory personnel (Price 1977, pp. 37-38), there is strong reason to believe that the supervisory nurses will be quite different from the nonsupervisory nurses.

Registered nurses with three types of training are employed by the hospitals: diploma (N=770, 71 percent), associate (N=140, 13 percent), and baccalaureate (N=174, 13 percent).[4] The diploma nurses are hospital-trained for three years, the associate nurses attend two-year community colleges, and the baccalaureate nurses are the products of four-year courses in colleges and universities. Based on comparisons with national statistics, the diploma nurses in our sample are overrepresented, whereas the associate and baccalaureate nurses are underrepresented (Anderson 1968, p. 9). The trend in the United States is for the long-term growth of the baccalaureate type of training and the decline of the diploma and associate types of training.

To expand on our discussion in Chapter 1, we offer five reasons for studying registered nurses. (1) They are the most responsible health professional whose presence in the hospital is continuous. The contrast of registered nurses with physicians and licensed practical nurses is instructive. Physicians have more training than the nurses, but they spend very little time in the hospital. Licensed practical nurses, on the other hand, are continuously in the hospital, but they lack the training possessed by the nurses. Nurses, therefore, constitute critically important personnel in caring for patients in voluntary, short-term general hospitals.

(2) Registered nurses have comparatively high rates of turnover. As indicated in the first chapter, occupations comparable to nurses in training and sex composition, such as teachers and social workers, have considerably lower turnover rates than nurses. Given nurses' critical role in patient care in hospitals, these high rates of nursing turnover pose a serious threat to the maintenance of quality care for patients; the high rate of nursing turnover also means that provision of a given level of care is more costly to the hospital than would be the case with less turnover. In brief, the high rates of nursing turnover threaten hospital effectiveness and productivity.[5]

(3) Nurses are studied because of their professional status. There is, of course, research on nursing turnover.[6] The work of Kramer (1968, 1969, 1974, Kramer and Baker 1971) and Brief (1976) has already been mentioned. However, most of the research on turnover has focused on blue-collar occupations, where turnover has been greatest (Farris 1971; Lefkowitz 1971, p. 85; Ronan 1967). Among the white-collar occupations which have been studied, the study of professionals has been especially neglected, primarily because their turnover has not usually been large (Price 1977, p. 57). The study of nurses thus offers an opportunity to provide data about a relatively neglected type of occupation, professional employees.

(4) Most nurses are women. Lysaught, in a recent study of nursing and nursing education, states (1970, p. 33) that "approximately ninety-nine percent of the registered nurses in active practice are women." Since men have traditionally filled blue-collar occupations, the primary focus on these occupations in previous research means that most of the turnover research has focused on men. Our research should thus provide an opportunity to assess the findings of a causal model based mostly on data collected for men.

(5) Finally, nurses are selected because a significant proportion of them are part-time employees. Glaser points out (Davis 1966, p. 40) that "over two-fifths of American hospital general duty nurses are now part-time." In our research, 38 percent of the nurses are part-time employees. Since most of the blue-collar men traditionally studied are full-time employees, the result has been a relative neglect of part-time employees. Our research will consequently contribute data about a neglected segment of the labor force, part-time employees.[7] In addition, since part-time workers are becoming more important in the labor force—their percentage of the labor force increased from 11 to 14 between 1965 and 1970 (U.S. Bureau of

Labor Statistics 1975, p. 75)—it becomes even more necessary to examine this category of worker.

Nursing is, in brief, a strategic occupation to study. Nurses constitute a critical occupational category in an important part of the health-care-delivery system in the United States; have comparatively high rates of turnover, and, therefore, threaten the effectiveness and productivity of voluntary, short-term general hospitals; and are a professional occupation consisting mostly of females with a sizable contingent of part-time employees, thereby providing an opportunity to study workers who have heretofore been relatively neglected in the study of turnover. Few occupations provide so many advantages to study as that of the registered nurse.

DATA COLLECTION

Data collection extended over a period of approximately 23 months. Four fairly distinct periods can be distinguished.

The first period—January and February of 1976—involved obtaining permission to study the seven hospitals. Most of the time and effort during this period was devoted to describing the proposed research to managerial personnel in the hospitals, mostly nursing directors and first-level supervisors. All of the hospitals approached agreed to participate in the research.

The second period—March, April, and May of 1976—was primarily concerned with preparation of a questionnaire to administer to the nurses. A concerted effort was made to discuss the questionnaire with all supervisory personnel, especially the first-level nursing supervisors. Personnel officers were also sometimes involved in these discussions.

Prior to this research, Price (Price and Bluedorn 1979) had conducted a field study of the determinants of nursing turnover in another voluntary, short-term general hospital. Some nurses from this earlier study consented to serve as respondents to pretest the questionnaire used to collect the data for our research. The final questionnaire which emerged was a modified version of the questionnaire which Price had used in his previous research. Appendix A, at the end of the book, contains a copy of the questionnaire which we used in this research.

The questionnaire was distributed during the third period of data collection, which extended from June 1976 through August 1976. In June 1976 the hospitals were requested to supply the names and addresses of their nonsupervisory registered nurses. The final list consisted of 1,383 nurses, who were to receive the questionnaires.

In July 1976, written notices describing the research were distributed to all hospital personnel through hospital newsletters and to the nonsupervisory registered nurses through memoranda and fact sheets to all nursing units. These written notices contained information about the proposed research and about the researchers.[8]

Questionnaires were mailed to most of the 1,383 nurses in August 1976. Since one hospital had declined to supply the addresses of its nurses, questionnaires were distributed to these nurses by a research assistant on the project when they picked up their paychecks. All questionnaires—those mailed and those distributed with the paychecks—were to be returned to the researchers at the University of Iowa. A total of 1,101 questionnaires were returned, for a response rate of 80 percent. Such a response rate is quite high (Heberlein and Baumgartner 1978) for mailed questionnaires and signifies a strong motivation to cooperate in the research project. Not only should strongly motivated respondents provide valid and reliable data, but the response rate should result in limited, if any, selection bias. The high degree of nursing cooperation was, at least partly, the result of the splendid cooperation of the hospital administrators, especially of those from the nursing departments. Table 3-2 indicates the distribution and receipt of the questionnaires by hospital.

Table 3-2: Questionnaire Distribution and Returns, by Hospital

Hospital	Questionnaires Distributed	Questionnaires Returned	Percentage Returned
1	126	93	74
2[a]	147	114	78
3	202	165	82
4	272	199	75
5	216	175	81
6	289	239	83
7	134	116	87
TOTAL	1,383	1,101	80

[a] Hospital 2 declined to supply the addresses of its nurses.

The fourth and final period consisted of collection of the turnover data. In September 1977, each hospital received a list of the nurses who had returned the questionnaires, and was requested to indicate the names of all nurses no longer employed by the hospital as of October 1, 1977. As well as the nurses no longer employed, the hospitals were also requested to indicate those who had died, retired, or were dismissed. This information was collected by a visit to each hospital in October 1977. Approximately fourteen months had transpired between distribution of the questionnaires and collection of the turnover data.

Each list was cross-checked with at least two individuals during the visit to a hospital, mostly with knowledgeable persons in the nursing departments (directors, assistant directors, and secretaries). In several instances, however, individuals in the personnel departments (directors and/or their secretaries) supplied critical information.

Two slight changes were made as a result of the cross-checks. Several nurses had resigned because of serious physical illness, such as heart attacks. Where such illnesses could be clearly verified, these nurses were classified as involuntary turnover and were removed from the analysis. The second change involved nurses who intended to resign. Some of the nurses still employed by the hospital in September intended to resign by October 1, 1977. When these nurses had submitted letters of resignation, they were counted as quits. A later telephone check with the hospitals indicated that these nurses had quit.

The collection of the turnover data resulted in two categories of nurses. First, those who had left employment of the hospitals or had submitted a letter of resignation since they returned the questionnaires in the Fall of 1976. There were 221 of these "leavers," or 20 percent of the sample. The second category of nurse consisted of those who were still employed by the hospitals. There were 880 of these "stayers," or 80 percent of the sample. The questionnaires collected from the nurses in August 1976 were matched with the turnover data collected in October 1977 by means of numbers on the face sheet of the questionnaires. Each nurse was, of course, informed about the existence and purpose of the number.[9]

In the first chapter we indicated that this research was concerned with voluntary turnover. Therefore, from the 221 leavers were subtracted the number of nurses who left involuntarily because of death, retirement, dismissal, or serious physical disability. Ten nurses left involuntarily, or 1 percent of the sample. These ten nurses were dropped from the analysis, thereby reducing the N from 1,101 to 1,091.

The essential task of the analysis is to indicate, based on the causal model, the significant differences between the voluntary leavers (19 percent of the sample) and the stayers (80 percent of the sample).[10] In this research, as noted in the first chapter, the study of turnover involves a study of leavers and stayers. The stayers must be studied because they are essential as a basis of comparison with the leavers. Turnover in our research thus does not mean an exclusive focus on leavers, as it does in some research.

Research on nurses commonly finds a much higher percentage of involuntary turnover than the 1 percent we found in our research (Eaton 1968, p. 88; Lyons 1970; Wieland 1969). Lyons, for instance, who has done significant work on nursing turnover, notes (p. 74) that about two-thirds of nursing turnover is typically involuntary. The reason involuntary turnover is so low in our research is that we classify as voluntary turnover all nurses who resign because of kinship responsibilities, such as having a baby or moving to a new community because of a change in the spouse's job. Since many nurses leave because of kinship responsibilities, classification of these nurses as involuntary turnovers—as is done in much research on nursing turnover—results in a much higher percentage of involuntary turnover. In our opinion, nurses who leave because of kinship responsibilities are making a choice: they are assigning greater priority to kinship roles than to occupational roles. And such choices are the essential ingredient of what is commonly meant by voluntary turnover. Table 3-3 presents, by hospital, the turnover data just described.

Table 3-3: Turnover Data, by Hospital

Hospital	Stayers		Voluntary Leaving		Involuntary Leaving	
	N	Percent	N	Percent	N	Percent
1	75	80.6	17	18.3	1	1.1
2	91	79.8	21	18.4	2	1.8
3	135	84.2	26	15.8	0	0.0
4	148	74.4	51	25.6	0	0.0
5	148	84.6	26	14.9	1	.6
6	201	84.1	37	15.5	1	.4
7	78	67.2	33	28.4	5	4.3
TOTAL	880	79.9	211	19.2	10	.9

One final note is necessary on data collection. The nurses were not asked to state verbally their "reasons for leaving." Such reasons are often obtained from nurses by hospitals during exit interviews and placed in the records. Many researchers make use of these records when studying the determinants of turnover; the reasons for leaving, as stated by the nurses and recorded by the hospital, become the determinants of turnover. This type of data collection has been justifiably criticized because of the poor quality of information obtained (Hinrichs 1971, 1975; Lefkowitz and Katz 1969; Smith and Kerr 1953). Respondents in exit interviews, for instance, are unlikely to criticize the hospital for fear of jeopardizing future employment, and often "rationalize" their account of why they are leaving.

It is important to reiterate that our study is based on longitudinal data and does not make use of verbally stated reasons for leaving. In August 1976, the nurses were asked, by questionnaire, to describe themselves and their situations; these descriptions pertained to variables which previous research had indicated as possible determinants of turnover. In October 1977, based on data collected by means of records and interviews within the hospitals, these nurses were classified as either leavers or stayers. It is the task of the analysis, as previously indicated, to see if the leavers and stayers differ significantly on the personal and situational characteristics measured in the questionnaire.

MEASUREMENT

The measures used for all of the variables in our model are presented in Appendix B at the end of the book. We were at a distinct advantage in developing these measures because of the prior measurement work of Price (1972a) and the previously cited field study of nursing turnover in a voluntary, short-term general hospital (Price and Bluedorn 1979). Because of this, the majority of the items used to form the indices had previously been used and have been accepted as valid and reliable. However, even with this assurance that our measures are appropriate by social science standards, we conducted a number of the checks typically used to evaluate measurement validity and reliability.

Validity was assessed in three ways. First, using factor analysis on nine of the variables, we determined whether the items selected to measure a particular variable formed a single factor with high factor loadings. Finding this can be interpreted to mean the items measure the same underlying construct and can be combined into a single index. This type of validity has been referred to as "convergent validity," which is a form of construct validity (Bohrnstedt 1970; Campbell and Fiske 1959). Second, we determined the degree of interrcorrelation among the indices obtained in the above manner. This procedure is often used to assess what is referred to as "discriminant validity"–the expectation is that measures of different constructs should not be highly correlated. We certainly did not expect our indices to be uncorrelated with one another, however. There is a tremendous volume of formal organization literature on how the characteristics of organizations are interrelated. For example, we expect variables such as routinization, participation, instrumental communication, and so on to be correlated at a low to moderate level. In addition, our causal model shows that we expect turnover, job satisfaction, and intent to stay to be causally influenced by the other variables in the model. Thus, we expect these dependent variables to be at least moderately correlated with the variables hypothesized to be causally antecedent. If, however, the indices we use are highly intercorrelated, then we would have to conclude that these measures do not adequately discriminate among the constructs we wish to measure–the measures we use overlap too much, and we will not be able to determine the influence of the separate constructs. Finally, for the measures which could not be evaluated with factor analysis, we relied primarily on their "face" validity as well as on their discriminant validity and, in one instance, predictive validity.

The reliability of our measures will be assessed, when possible, by measuring the internal consistency among the items composing the index. We use Cronbach's Alpha (1951), the reliability coefficient commonly used for this purpose.

The questionnaire included multiple items intended to measure the following nine variables: opportunity, job satisfaction, routinization, participation, instrumental communication, professionalism, integration, distributive justice, and promotional opportunity. As already indicated, most of these items were based on previous measurement work by Price (1972a), but especially helpful was the pilot study of a voluntary, short-term general hospital (Price and Bluedorn 1979).

The items for each of these nine variables were subjected to factor analysis (RAO initial-factoring method with varimax rotation).[11] Emergence of a single factor for a variable—which occurred for every variable except participation—was interpreted as evidence for the existence of a single dimension for the variable. Items whose loadings were low (a cutoff of approximately .40 was used) relative to other items for a variable were not used to construct the indices. For participation, where two factors emerged, one factor seemed to refer to more of the core elements of the concept, to have higher loadings, and to contain more items; this factor was thus selected to measure participation.

Table 3-4 indicates the number of items and average loadings of the items for the nine indices, and Appendix B reports the factor loadings for each item. The average loading of .75 is quite high, giving us added confidence that the items we selected on the basis of other research can validly be used to measure the constructs in our model. The indices used in the analysis are composites obtained by summing the scores on the items selected on the basis of factor analysis. These are commonly referred to as "factor-based scales" (Kim and Mueller 1978).

Table 3-4: Number of Items and Average Loadings for Nine Indices

Variables	Number of Items	Loadings
Opportunity	4	.63
Job Satisfaction	7	.87
Routinization	4	.71
Participation	4	.73
Instrumental Communication	7	.74
Integration	4	.73
Distributive Justice	3	.68
Promotional Opportunity	8	.78
Professionalism	3	.66
AVERAGE	4.88	.75

Table 3-5 presents a correlation matrix for all of the variables used in in the study. As may be seen by examining the correlations of these nine factor-based scales, among themselves and with other variables, none of the correlations is large. This may be interpreted as support for the discriminant validity of these measures.

Measures for the remaining four variables were not constructed and evaluated by factor analysis. These four variables, plus the number of questionnaire items used in their construction, are as follows: intent to stay (two items), pay (one item), general training (one item), and kinship responsibility (three items). These measures are accepted on the basis of their face validity and, as will be discussed below, on the basis of their predictive capacity or discriminatory power.

The two intent-to-stay items were combined into an index and assessed for predictive capacity by their ability to predict future turnover.[12] The estimate of what to expect comes from the previously cited field study (Price and Bluedorn 1979), where a correlation coefficient of -.50 was obtained between this index and turnover. Although a somewhat smaller coefficient (-.40) is found for our data, we are satisfied that this measure adequately captures the construct. In addition, an examination of Table 3-5 indicates that our measure correlates .30 or less with the other mea-

Table 3-5: Correlation Matrix for All Variables[a]

	1	2	3	4	5	6	7	8	9	10	11	12	13	14	15	16
1.	-															
2.	-.404	-														
3.	-.121	.300	-													
4.	.187	-.169	-.031	-												
5.	.005	-.063	-.374	-.039	-											
6.	-.044	.117	.238	.139	-.130	-										
7.	-.074	.145	.293	.056	-.108	.313	-									
8.	-.011	.035	.060	.014	-.072	.074	.089	-								
9.	.017	-.007	-.072	.063	.047	.016	.076	.167	-							
10.	-.025	.046	.060	-.033	-.039	-.046	-.003	.008	-.044	-						
11.	-.022	.102	.269	.086	-.188	.159	.128	.024	-.045	.163	-					
12.	.003	.022	.004	.060	-.126	.011	.052	.125	.142	-.068	-.021	-				
13.	.180	-.257	-.015	.191	-.016	-.003	-.095	-.032	.136	-.025	.020	-.010	-			
14.	-.110	.229	.103	-.132	-.002	-.002	.015	-.171	-.361	.025	-.029	-.066	-.292	-		
15.	.010	-.058	-.121	.069	.043	-.002	.011	.178	.781	-.084	-.023	.105	.151	-.437	-	
16.	-.190	.287	.123	-.172	.046	.028	.040	-.176	-.110	-.024	-.008	.034	-.235	.351	-.191	-
17.	-.223	.355	.074	-.226	-.018	.051	.161	-.007	-.109	.001	-.078	.016	-.341	.329	-.206	.596

[a]Pairwise N's used to compute the correlations range from 1,010 to 1,091.

Note: 1=Turnover: 2=Intent to Stay: 3=Job Satisfaction: 4=Opportunity: 5=Routinization: 6=Participation: 7=Instrumental Communication: 8=Integration: 9=Pay: 10=Distributive Justice: 11=Promotional Opportunity: 12=Professionalism: 13=General Training: 14=Kinship Responsibility: 15=Amount of Time Worked: 16=Age: 17=Length of Service.

sures, which are supposed to be conceptually distinct. In short, it has discriminant validity.

Pay is measured by a single questionnaire item and is accepted on the basis of face validity and discriminant validity; it is not highly correlated with the other variables (see Table 3-5).

General training, like pay, is measured by a single questionnaire item. Most nurses have been trained in hospital programs as diploma nurses. Only recently have associate (community college) and baccalaureate (university and college) types of training emerged. Since type of training is the questionnaire item used to measure general training—the diploma training being the most specific and the baccalaureate being the most general—the older and more experienced nurses should exhibit less of the more recent training than the younger and less experienced nurses. An examination of Table 3-5 indicates that the predicted patterns exist: general training and age = -.24 and general training and length of service = -.34. In addition, the indicator for general training is not strongly related to any of the other twelve determinants of turnover. All of the coefficients are below .30 (Table 3-5). Since general training is intended to be conceptually different from the other determinants, these low coefficients indicate adequate discriminant validity for the indicator.

Kinship responsibility is measured by an index based on information from three items. Since two of the items pertain to marriage and the existence of children, the older and more experienced nurses would be predicted to score higher on the index than the younger and less experienced nurses. An examination of Table 3-5 reveals that these predicted patterns, though relatively low, exist (kinship responsibility and age = .35 and kinship responsibility and length of service = .33). Kinship responsibility, as would be expected with acceptable discriminant validity, is not highly related to the other twelve determinants of turnover (Table 3-5).

Reliability of ten of the indices was assessed, as previously indicated, by Cronbach's coefficient Alpha (1951). Since pay and general training were measured by single items, and kinship responsibility was not obtained by simply summing items, an Alpha cannot be computed and used to assess the reliability of their measures. Table 3-6, which contains the Alphas for the ten indices, indicates that none of these falls below .74, and their average is .83. Since Nunnally (1967) recommends (p. 226) an Alpha of .80 for basic research, the ten indices appear to possess satisfactory internal consistency.

Table 3-7 contains the means and standard deviations for the measures of the thirteen concepts of the causal model. Since these measures are not standardized across studies, these statistics should not be compared with the results of other research. (Table 3-7 also contains the means and standard deviations for the nursing units, a topic to be discussed in the next section.)

One final measurement issue requires discussion. The preceding discussion has indicated that the thirteen determinants of the causal model are measured by individual perceptions and assessments as recorded on the questionnaires administered to the nurses. Individual perceptions pose relatively few problems as measures for intent to stay and job satisfaction since these two concepts refer to internal orientations of individuals; they are social psychological concepts which can properly be measured by an individual's response to clearly stated questions. The remaining eleven determinants, however, refer to individual behavior or situational conditions, and there is some question as to whether these are adequately measured by individual perceptions. Use of individual perceptions becomes even more problematic because we do not have other data, such as observations and records, to cross-check the questionnaires.

Table 3-6: Cronbach's Alpha for Ten Indices

Variables	Coefficient Alpha[a]
Intent to Stay	.85
Job Satisfaction	.87
Opportunity	.75
Routinization	.82
Centralization	.86
Instrumental Communication	.90
Integration	.84
Distributive Justice	.76
Promotional Opportunity	.93
Professionalism	.74
AVERAGE	.83

[a]Standardized-item Alpha.

Table 3-7: Variable Means and Standard Deviations for Individuals and Nursing Units

Variables	Individual		Nursing Units	
	Mean	SD	Mean	SD
Turnover	.19	.40	.20	.12
Intent to Stay	6.39	2.05	6.37	.76
Job Satisfaction	28.26	4.03	28.29	1.81
Opportunity	11.40	2.70	11.24	1.07
Routinization	11.93	2.92	12.08	1.68
Participation	13.89	3.46	10.35	1.56
Instrumental Communication	26.37	5.04	26.42	2.00
Integration	8.52	5.28	8.79	1.92
Pay	$8,455	$3,027	$8,802	$1,494
Distributive Justice	7.01	1.63	6.99	.65
Promotional Opportunity	21.62	6.07	21.40	2.95
Professionalism	1.79	1.36	1.92	.72
General Training	1.45	.75	1.30	.26
Kinship Responsibility	4.88	1.34	4.91	.53
	(N=1091)		(N=63)	

There is no denying the difficulty of measuring behavior and situational conditions by the reports of respondents. Three justifications are offered for the use of these measures. First, organizational researchers typically measure these characteristics by individual perceptions collected by questionnaires and/or interviews. Price's review (1972a) of the state of organizational measurement clearly indicates the widespread use of individual perceptions to measure behavioral and situational concepts.[13] Our approach is thus in conformity with current procedures of organizational research. The second justification for the measurement approach of our research is that for the checks that are available to us, we find adequate validity for all of the indices. The nine indices constructed on the basis of previous research and evaluated by means of factor analysis are our most adequate measures. Finally, and as a preview of our findings, the results of our research are in basic agreement with the causal model.

Since the model is intended to be a plausible summary of the turnover literature, this means that our research agrees with what other scholars have found about the determinants of turnover. The case for our measurement approach would be seriously weakened without this agreement with prior research. Improvement of the level of organizational measurement is a long-term task, and we feel that we have moved forward a little in the direction of improved measurement.[14]

DATA ANALYSIS

The primary focus of this section is on the statistical procedures (multiple regression and path analysis) used to analyze the data. First, however, it is necessary to discuss briefly the issues of "missing values" and "units of analysis."

Respondents who do not supply complete data pose a problem when multivariate analysis is the goal. Less confidence, for example, can be placed in the results when the amount of missing data is high. In such situations, there is serious concern that the respondents who did not answer the questions might be systematically different from those who responded to the questions. This situation is further complicated by the fact that the size of the N constantly changes when different variables have varying degrees of missing values. The issue of missing values must therefore be faced.

The primary concern with missing data is for the nurses who did not return the questionnaires (282 nurses). Although we do not have background data on these nurses which could be used to determine how they differ from the 80 percent of the nurses who did return the questionnaire, it is possible to make some assessment of whether they comprise a unique subsample. Because we used hospital records to measure turnover, it was possible to compute the turnover rate of these 282 nurses. Their rate was .28, as compared to .20 for those who returned the questionnaires. This suggests limited, if any, bias associated with not including these nurses in the analysis.

Table 3-8 indicates the missing cases for the thirteen determinants in the causal model. The average number and percentage of missing cases are, respectively, twenty-four and two. Even where these values are the highest–forty-five and four for promotional opportunity–the magnitudes are not large enough to introduce complications into the analysis. Since the turnover data were collected directly from the seven hospitals, there are no missing cases for the key dependent variable.[15]

Two units of analysis are used. The bulk of our analysis uses individuals as the unit. Individual measures of the thirteen determinants are used to assess individual differences in those who stay and leave. This is consistent with most of the previous research on turnover; social psychologists have provided much of the turnover data, and they use the individual as the unit of analysis. The N for this part of our analysis is 1,091.

We also collected data about the nursing units to which the nurses were assigned. Since the seven hospitals were basically alike, they had many similar nursing units. If a unit had five or more nurses, it was considered large enough for use in the analysis. Sixty-three units met this criterion, and these units contain 72 percent of the nurses in the sample. When the nursing unit is used as the unit of analysis, all variables in the causal model, including turnover, use pooled measures. The results for the individuals in the unit are summed (aggregated) and a mean calculated; this mean then becomes the score for the unit. For turnover, the rate of voluntary leaving is used as the unit score. A fair amount of turnover research

Table 3-8: Missing Cases for Each Variable

Variables	Number of Missing Cases	Percentage of Missing Cases[a]
Intent to Stay	15	01
Job Satisfaction	20	02
Opportunity	35	03
Routinization	13	01
Participation	39	04
Instrumental Communication	20	02
Integration	8	01
Pay	19	02
Distributive Justice	27	02
Promotional Opportunity	45	04
Professionalism	29	03
General Training	7	01
Kinship Responsibility	30	03
AVERAGE	23.6	02

[a]This percentage is figured on an N of 1,091 because the ten examples of involuntary turnover are excluded from this analysis.

uses some form of social system as its unit, especially the research performed by sociologists. Table 3-7 presents the means and standard deviations for the variables and the two units of analysis. (We also undertake analysis of the hospital as the unit of analysis in Chapter 7. These data are found in Appendix 7-2.)

Most research does not use both the individual and the social unit in data analysis; the customary pattern is to use one or the other unit of analysis. We believe that our research is unique because the causal model will be estimated for both units of analysis.

The data are analyzed by multiple-regression and path-analytic techniques. Multiple-regression analysis is useful for this research because it allows for an assessment of the net influence of each variable relative to the others, as well as for an indication of the total explanatory power of the model. (1) Prior research on turnover has indicated that the variables in the causal model are probable determinants of turnover. However, since this prior research has not generally controlled for the possible influence of all significant determinants, it is impossible to know if a determinant's influence is nonspurious and which determinants are the most important. Multiple regression, because it provides standardized net coefficients, is a particularly useful technique for this purpose. (2) We especially want to estimate the total explanatory power of the model because we have sought to include in the model all major determinants of turnover. It is our hope that with our comprehensive model we can increase the amount of explained variance for turnover.

The causal model, as described in Chapter 2, shows both direct and indirect influences on turnover. Intent to stay, for instance, is believed to have a direct impact on turnover, whereas the impact of job satisfaction on turnover is believed to be indirect, through intent to stay. All of the determinants in our model, with the exception of intent to stay and opportunity, are hypothesized to have indirect effects on turnover. Path analysis is a statistical technique which allows for estimating direct, indirect, and total effects for the variables in the model (Land 1969; Heise 1969; Duncan 1966).

The use of multiple-regression and path-analytic techniques involves assumptions about the model to be tested and the nature of the data collected to test the model; the extent to which our research meets these assumptions is discussed in the notes which accompany the chapter.[16]

One final comment is necessary about the correlates of turnover. Our discussion of the model indicated that the correlates were excluded because they did not indicate how their effects on turnover were produced. Age was used for illustrative purposes when the correlates were discussed. There was no reason, as may be recalled, to include age in the model, since the variables which change with increasing age, and which are believed to produce effects on turnover, are already included in the model. As previously indicated, these variables were as follows: routinization, centralization, instrumental communication, integration, pay, and kinship responsibility. It is possible, however, that the model does not include all the turnover-relevant variables which change with increasing age. Many changes occur as employees become older, and it is possible that some of the changes may influence turnover and not be incorporated in the variables of the existing research. To check this possibility, the correlates can be introduced in the final stage of the regression analysis. Age and length of service will be the correlates used for this purpose since they are the ones found in most literature. Whenever addition of these variables significantly increases the explained variance, we will interpret it to mean that the model has failed to indicate fully the variables which produce variations in turnover and which also are correlated with age and/or length of service.

The correlates can be used in another important way in the analysis. It is possible that the causal model does not accurately portray the influence of the determinants for all categories of nurses. The prior field work conducted by Price, for instance, indicated a strong belief among hospital administrators that full-time and part-time nurses were very different.[17] Data collection for the current research, although it was not accompanied by as intensive a field study as was Price's prior study, also indicated that the hospital administrators believed that major differences characterized the full-time and part-time nurses.

Amount of time worked, whether full-time or part-time, is a correlate like age and length of service. To check the causal model separately for full-time and part-time nurses is to check for what statisticians term "interaction effects" (Kerlinger and Pedhazur 1973, pp. 181-182). The literature about organizations commonly refers to this type of approach–the checking of interaction effects–as "contingency theory."[18] In organizational terms, this approach means that there is no "one best way" to structure an organization to decrease turnover: what works for full time nurses, for instance, may not work for part-time nurses. Contingency theory represents a criticism of classical management theory, as embodied, for example, in the work of Frederick W. Taylor.[19]

Our analysis will check the model separately for the full-time and part-time nurses. Since age and length of service are so important in the turnover literature, the model will also be checked for interactions with these correlates. Three correlates are thus used to check for interaction effects–amount of time worked, age, and length of service–and represent our use of the contingency approach.[20]

The problem has been described, the causal model has been explicated, and the methodology indicated. What remains now is to present the results of the research, and it is to this task that we now turn.

NOTES

1. This size classification for hospitals comes from Becker and Neuhauser (1975, p. 99).

2. Hospitals, of course, also depend on the physicians for patient referral.

3. We also suspect that turnover has a greater negative impact on the effectiveness and productivity of service organizations. The quality of personal relationships, for example, seems to be somewhat less important in goods-producing organizations than in service-producing organizations. We can conceive of mines and factories which are very profitable and productive but which have relatively poor personal relationships. It is difficult for us to conceive of a university which does a very good job of teaching and research while simultaneously experiencing relatively poor personal relationships, especially between the faculty and the students. What would be true for universities would also be true for other service organizations, especially those which are mostly staffed by professionals (hospitals, law firms, laboratories, and so forth). We know of no evidence to support our suspicions, however.

4. This total does not add to 1,091 because seven nurses did not answer the question about type of training. The small number of nurses with graduate training is included in our category of "baccalaureate nurse."

5. As the first chapter indicates, the high rates of nursing turnover are important for reasons other than their impact on hospital effectiveness and productivity. However, since most of the literature which examines the impact of nursing turnover on hospitals focuses on effectiveness and productivity, we have emphasized these two outcomes.

6. For an indication of this literature, see Price (1977, pp. 141-154).

7. Gannon (Gannon and Nothern 1971; Gannon and Brainin 1971) is one of the few scholars who has examined the turnover of part-time employees.

8. Key parts of this information were also contained on the face sheet of our questionnaire. (See Appendix A.)

9. The idea to use numbers for purposes of identification was suggested to us by researchers at the Survey Research Center of the University of Michigan. Not only were the nurses informed about the existence and purpose of the number, but they were free to return or not to return the questionnaires. In short, the nurses were subjected to no coercion by the hospitals or the researchers. We did not even send out the customary follow-up note (mostly because of expense) to nurses who did not return the questionnaire.

10. We ignore the 1 percent of the nurses who were involuntary leavers.

11. See Kim and Mueller (1978) for a discussion of factor analysis.

12. One of these items is from the work of Lyons (1968) on nurses, whereas the other is from the National Opinion Research Center (1972) study of priests.

13. These behavioral concepts are often termed "structural" characteristics of organizations.

14. We could, of course, redefine our concepts to make them refer to subjective orientations. With this approach, opportunity, for example, rather than being "the availability of alternate jobs in the organization's environment," becomes instead "the perceived availability." This approach makes little sense to us because the literature reviewed for our causal model generally refers to objective characteristics rather than to subjective orientations.

15. See Kim and Curry (1977) for a complete treatment of missing-data

problems.

16. Multiple-regression analysis has traditionally been presented as requiring variables measured at an interval level. With the exception of turnover, most of the variables in our causal model are measured at the ordinal level. Contemporary literature, however, suggests that multiple-regression analysis can and should be used with ordinal-level independent variables (Labovitz 1967, 1970; Kim 1975).

Multiple-regression analysis assumes linearity between the independent and dependent variables. If this requirement is not met, the data typically are transformed to produce a linear relationship. In this research, however, transformations are less suitable because most of the variables are measured at the ordinal level. The analysis also becomes unmanageable with transformations. Since job satisfaction, intent to stay, and turnover are treated as dependent variables at various stages in the analysis, transformations would result in the same variable being estimated at one stage as transformed and at another stage as untransformed. Most important, however, we have empirical evidence that nonlinearity is not a serious problem. We transformed all independent variables into sets of dummy variables and conducted regression analysis on these sets to determine if substantial additional explained variance, over and above that obtained for the interval-level variables, is obtained. Regressing job satisfaction on all causally prior variables produces an increase of .016; regressing intent to stay on all causally prior variables produces an increase of .029; and regressing turnover on all causally prior variables produces an increase of .036. From this we conclude there is very little nonlinearity in our model and our findings will be only trivially biased by any nonlinearity which is present.

Use of multiple regression assumes additive relationships among the variables in the equation. As described in the text, we will test for the presence of interactions and take appropriate steps if they are found.

Multiple-regression analysis assumes no substantial intercorrelations among the independent variables. If they exist, we have what is referred to as the problem of "multicollinearity," which can result in estimation and interpretation difficulties (Gordon 1968). Although the pilot study (Price and Bluedorn 1979) indicated that this would not be a problem in this research, we will examine the zero-order correlations to assess this possibility.

Application of multiple regression requires the equivalence of variances for the dependent variable for various levels of an independent variable, that is, homoscedasticity. Because the major dependent variable of this research is a dichotomy (leavers and stayers), this assumption is violated. However, recent literature (Knoke 1975; Goodman 1976; Gillespie 1977) indicates that violation of this assumption is not serious when the proportions in the two categories are not extreme, that is, when the split is approximately 75 percent and 25 percent. Use of signficance tests with multiple regression also requires that the dependent variable be normally distributed at various levels of the independent variable. This is also a problem when the dependent variable is a dichotomy. However, given the reasonable split on this variable in this research, and given that tests of statistical significance are used primarily to reduce arbitrariness in the inferences drawn from the data, any violations are assumed to have only minor effects on the conclusions. (Technically speaking, this is research on the entire population rather than on a sample.)

17. Gannon's research (Gannon and Nothern 1971) also indicates that full-time workers and part-time workers are very different.

18. For an excellent review and critique of the contingency approach, see Schoonhoven (1977). For more detailed information, see also Galbraith

(1973), Lawrence and Lorsch (1969), and Woodward (1965).

19. See Aitken (1960) for an excellent description of the Taylor approach to scientific management.

20. Also relevant is the work of Farrell (1978) and Katz (1978).

CHAPTER 4
Correlational Data

The results of our research will be presented in the next four chapters. This chapter presents the results without controls, that is, the relationships between the determinants and turnover are examined without statistically removing the effects of the other variables in the causal model. Such data, often referred to as "zero-order" or "bivariate" results, will serve as an introduction to the more complicated results produced by our "multivariate analysis" using multiple-regression and path-analytic techniques. The fifth and sixth chapters will present these multivariate results when the data are analyzed with the individual as the unit of analysis. Finally, the seventh chapter will present the results where the immediate work group, the nursing unit, is used to analyze the data. Both zero-order and multivariate data for the nursing units will be presented in the seventh chapter.

ZERO-ORDER COEFFICIENTS FOR INDIVIDUALS

Although turnover is the dependent variable of our research, application of path analysis to our causal model requires that job satisfaction, intent to stay, and turnover be viewed successively as "dependent" variables. This use of path analysis will be illustrated in the next three chapters. Table 4-1 presents the zero-order coefficients for the independent variables with each of these three dependent variables. These coefficients are Pearson product-moment correlation coefficients and indicate the degree of association between the two variables without holding constant the influence of other variables. If a correlation between two variables is equal to or less than $|\pm .06|$ in Table 4-1, then we will assume that the two variables are unrelated; correlation coefficients greater than $|\pm .06|$ are statistically significant at the .05 level.

Job Satisfaction

Six determinants of the model are related to job satisfaction by the statistical-significance criterion: routinization, instrumental communication, promotional opportunity, participation, kinship responsibility, and pay. All of these relationships are consistent with the causal model.

The model indicates that increased routinization is expected to depress job satisfaction; therefore, the negative zero-order coefficient for routin-

Table 4-1: Zero-Order Correlation Coefficients for the Entire Sample[a]

Independent Variables	Dependent Variables		
	Job Satisfaction	Intent to Stay	Turnover
Intent to Stay			-.40
Job Satisfaction		.30	-.12
Opportunity	-.03	-.17	.19
Routinization	-.37	-.06	.01
Participation	.24	.12	-.04
Instrumental Communication	.29	.15	-.07
Integration	.06	.04	-.01
Pay	.07	-.01	.02
Distributive Justice	.06	.05	-.03
Promotional Opportunity	.27	.10	-.02
Professionalism	.00	.02	.00
General Training	-.02	-.26	.18
Kinship Responsibility	.10	.23	-.11
Age	.12	.29	-.19
Length of Service	.07	.36	-.22
Amount of Time Worked	-.12	-.06	.01

[a]A coefficient > $|\pm .06|$ is statistically significant at $p < .05$.

ization is expected. Nurses whose jobs are repetitive express dissatisfaction with their work. The model also indicates that increases in instrumental communication, promotional opportunity, and participation are expected to result in greater job satisfaction; the three positive zero-order coefficients for these determinants thus are consistent with the model. Nurses who are well informed about their jobs, who have a good opportunity to get ahead occupationally in the hospital, and who make many decisions about their jobs are the nurses who like their work.

Kinship responsibility is expected to decrease turnover through intent to stay; no impact on job satisfaction is expected. Should an impact exist on job satisfaction, however–and such an impact is plausible–the impact should be positive, since this would reduce turnover in the expected manner. A positive correlation is found, that is, nurses with the greatest kinship responsibilities state that they like their jobs. The most important kinship responsibilities in our research are being married and having children. Finally, pay, based on the model, is expected to depress turnover by a positive impact on job satisfaction. The positive correlation which exists between pay and job satisfaction is thus expected: the nurses who receive more money are more satisfied with their jobs.

The three correlates–age, length of service, and amount of time worked–are also related to job satisfaction. Chapter 3 indicated two ways the correlates of turnover will be used to check our model: (1) to find out if our determinants account for variation normally attributed to the correlates, and (2) to see if the model differs for various categories of nurses, as defined by the correlates. To be used for this purpose, however, the relationships of the correlates with the determinants must be consistent with the turnover literature. Since age and length of service are generally negatively related to turnover–it is the older nurses with more seniority who less often leave the hospitals–it is expected that age and length of service will be positively related to job satisfaction. Only by increasing job satisfaction could age and length of service be negatively related to turnover. It is thus not surprising that the coefficients of age and length of service with job satisfaction are positive. It is the older nurses with more seniority who are more satisfied with their jobs. We will continue to treat age and length of service as separate correlates because even though they are fairly highly correlated (r = .60), they do not measure the same thing.

We have no expectations about the correlation between amount of time worked, whether full-time or part-time, and job satisfaction because there is no well-established relationship between these variables in the literature. We can only report that the part-time nurses exhibit greater job satisfaction than the full-time nurses.

The zero-order coefficients for routinization, instrumental communication, promotional opportunity, and participation with job satisfaction are substantially larger than the coefficients for kinship responsibility and pay. For routinization, as an illustration, the coefficient is almost four times as large as the coefficient for kinship responsibility and more than five times the coefficient for pay. These preliminary results are especially interesting because the importance of pay is supported by a very substantial body of research. Based only on the amount of supporting data from past research, we would have expected to find that pay was more strongly related to job satisfaction than any other determinant.

Five determinants do not meet our statistical-significance criterion: opportunity, integration, distributive justice, professionalism, and general training. Some of these determinants may, however, be related to the other two dependent variables to be treated, intent to stay and turnover. At this point, however, it must be noted that the zero-order coefficients indicate little potential causal significance for job opportunities outside the hospital, the existence of close friends within the hospital, the extent to which input into the hospital is linked to rewards and punishments, the dedication to professional standards of performance, and occupational socialization which increases the productivity of different hospitals.

Intent to Stay

Seven determinants have statistically significant coefficients with intent to stay: job satisfaction, general training, kinship responsibility, opportunity, instrumental communication, participation, and promotional opportunity.

These findings are all consistent with the relationships predicted by the model. Since the model indicates that job satisfaction and kinship responsibility are expected to increase intent to stay, the positive coefficients for these two determinants are expected. Nurses who are very satisfied with their jobs and who have many local kin express a strong likelihood of remaining in their jobs. Since the model indicates that general training is expected to decrease intent to stay, the negative coefficient for general training is also expected. Nurses with the most general type of training—baccalaureate training in our research—evidence weak intent to remain in their jobs.

The model indicates that instrumental communication, participation, and promotional opportunity are expected to have an impact on intent to stay through job satisfaction. Increases in each of these determinants are expected to increase job satisfaction, which, in turn, is expected to increase intent to stay. It is, however, expected that these three determinants are positively correlated with intent to stay when job satisfaction is not controlled. Nurses who are well informed about their jobs, who actively participate in making job-related decisions, and who have a good opportunity to advance occupationally in the hospital indicate that they intend to remain in their jobs. The multivariate analysis presented in the following chapters will allow us to examine these relationships again, but after other variables have been controlled.

Opportunity is expected, according to the model, to have a direct, positive impact on turnover. If it should be found that opportunity has an indirect impact on turnover through intent to stay–and such an impact is plausible–a negative impact on intent to stay would be expected, since this would result in more turnover. A negative correlation is found between opportunity and intent to stay; this correlation tells us that nurses who have many alternative jobs outside the hospital also indicate that they are likely to leave the hospital.

Two of our correlates, age and length of service, have statistically signficant coefficients. Since age and length of service are negatively related to turnover, positive coefficients would be expected, and are found, between these two correlates and intent to stay. Older nurses and those who have high seniority plan to remain in their jobs more often than younger nurses with low seniority.

The correlation coefficient for job satisfaction is larger than the coefficient for any other determinant. Its coefficient, for example, is twice the coefficient for instrumental communication and three times the coefficient for promotional opportunity. These preliminary results are informative because of the controversial role of job satisfaction as a determinant of turnover. As was previously indicated in the chapter on the causal model, the traditional importance assigned to job satisfaction recently has been questioned. Our findings, at this point, suggest that job satisfaction is probably an important determinant of turnover.

The coefficients for five determinants do not meet our statistical-significance criterion: routinization, integration, pay, distributive justice, and professionalism. The influence of these determinants, however, may be suppressed by other determinants; this possibility will be checked in the following two chapters.[1] Amount of time worked is the only correlate which is not significantly related to intent to stay.

Turnover

Six determinants are significantly related to turnover: intent to stay, opportunity, general training, job satisfaction, kinship responsibility, and instrumental communication. These relationships are all consistent with those indicated by the model.

Nurses who indicate that they intend to stay leave less often than nurses who indicate they intend to leave. As discussed in Chapter 2, we view intent to stay as one component of commitment as defined by Porter and his colleagues (Mowday et al. 1979). We may conclude, then, that high commitment to the hospital is predictive of low turnover. Nurses who have many alternative jobs available outside the hospital leave more often than nurses who have fewer opportunities. Job opportunity for nurses, it should be remembered, is not restricted to hospitals; they can also work for government agencies, business firms, schools, or in the offices of physicians in private practice.

Nurses with general training leave more often than nurses with more specific training. We have ordered, it may be recalled, the three types of nursing training, beginnning with the most general, as follows: baccalaureate, associate, and diploma. Baccalaureate nurses are trained in colleges and universities, associate nurses receive their training in community colleges, and diploma nurses are trained by the hospitals which employ them. Most nurses, as indicated previously, are trained as diploma nurses. Thus, from the positive correlation coefficient we may conclude that it is this dominant form of occupational socialization–"on-the-job" training leading to a diploma–which produces nurses least likely to leave the hospital.

Nurses who indicate that they are satisfied with their jobs leave less often than nurses who indicate less satisfaction with their jobs. Note that our model includes two types of social psychological concepts: an affective component (job satisfaction) and a cognitive component (intent to stay, a dimension of commitment). Most research on turnover has stressed job satisfaction and ignored intent to stay.

Nurses who evidence greater kinship responsibility leave less often than nurses with lesser kinship responsibility. This means that responsibilities associated with marriage and the care of children are positively related to keeping the nurses from quitting their jobs. Finally, instrumental communication and turnover are negatively related: the less the communication of job-related information to the nurses, the more their turnover.

Two correlates, age and length of service, have the expected negative relationships with turnover. Older nurses and those with more seniority exhibit less turnover than younger nurses and those with less seniority.

Intent to stay is more strongly related to turnover than any other determinant. Its coefficient is more than twice the size of the coefficient for opportunity, which is the second largest. Especially interesting is the fact that the coefficient for intent to stay is more than three times the coefficient for job satisfaction. Some of the scholars who criticize job satisfaction as a determinant of turnover, especially Porter and his colleagues (Mowday et al. 1979), posit commitment as a more important determinant of turnover than job satisfaction. Since we view intent to stay as a dimension of commitment, these preliminary findings appear to support the importance assigned to commitment by Porter and his colleagues. It may be recalled, however, that job satisfaction was more strongly related to intent to stay than any other determinant. These early results, therefore, appear to support commitment <u>and</u> job satisfaction as determinants of turnover. We will return to this topic again after the results of our multivariate analysis are presented.

The correlations for the following seven determinants do not meet the minimum statistical-significance criterion of greater than .06: participation, distributive justice, promotional opportunity, pay, integration, routinization, and professionalism. Four of these determinants–participation, promotional opportunity, pay, and routinization–were previously found to have been related to job satisfaction and/or intent to stay, thereby demonstrating some potential causal ordering significance for the later multivariate analysis. Distributive justice, integration, and professionalism, however, are not related to any of the dependent variables, thus raising doubts as to their causal significance. It is unlikely that determinants which are unrelated to job satisfaction, intent to stay, and turnover without control will later be related when net effects are examined. We shall not prematurely discard these three determinants, however. The multivariate analysis will allow us to determine whether there are suppressor effects operating.

MEANS FOR LEAVERS AND STAYERS

The material in the two previous sections has examined the zero-order coefficients for the entire sample of nurses. Another way to present the results without controls is to focus on the mean scores of the independent variables for the leavers and stayers. Table 4-2 contains the information to make these comparisons. The standard deviations are also included in the table, although we will not focus on them because we have no expec-

Table 4-2: Means and Standard Deviations of Leavers and Stayers for Entire Sample

Variables	Leavers		Stayers	
	Mean	S.D.	Mean	S.D.
Intent to Stay	4.69	2.10	6.79	1.82
Job Satisfaction	27.25	4.58	28.49	3.86
Opportunity	12.43	2.87	11.16	2.60
Routinization	11.96	2.97	11.92	2.91
Participation	13.58	3.50	13.96	3.45
Instrumental Communication	26.61	5.49	26.55	4.91
Integration	8.40	5.43	8.55	5.24
Pay	$8,562	$2,897	$8,429	$3,058
Distributive Justice	6.93	1.70	7.03	1.62
Promotional Opportunity	21.36	6.09	21.69	6.07
Professionalism	1.80	1.35	1.79	1.36
General Training	1.73	.88	1.38	.71
Kinship Responsibility	4.58	1.41	4.95	1.31
Age	27.43	7.81	32.54	10.98
Length of Service	2.51	1.13	3.24	1.29
Amount of Time Worked	.63	.48	.62	.49

tations about the variation of dispersion of the determinants for the leavers and stayers.

The causal model leads us to expect higher mean scores for the leavers for the following four determinants: opportunity, routinization, professionalism, and general training; that is, leavers should score higher than the stayers for alternative jobs outside the hospitals, repetitive work, dedication to professional standards, and general training. All differences in Table 4-2 are in the expected directions, although there is very little difference in the means for routinization and professionalism.

Lower mean scores for leavers are expected for the following nine determinants: intent to stay, job satisfaction, participation, instrumental communication, integration, pay, distributive justice, promotional opportunity, and kinship responsibility. The leavers should indicate less intent to stay, less satisfaction with their work, lower participation in decisions about their work, less receipt of work-related information, fewer close friends, less pay, less fairness in the distribution of pay, reduced opportunity to get ahead, and fewer local kin. Age and length of service should also have lower means for the leavers. Since there is little literature about the relationship between amount of time worked and turnover, we have no expectations for this correlate. With the exception of pay, all of the means in Table 4-2 are in the expected directions. There is, however, little difference in the means of the leavers and stayers for participation, integration, promotional opportunity, and kinship responsibilities.

DISCUSSION

All of the zero-order correlation coefficients are consistent with the causal model. Even the magnitudes of the coefficients are consistent with our expectations. The results at this stage in the analysis indicate that the following ten determinants are most important: intent to stay, job satisfaction, opportunity, general training, kinship responsibility, participation, instrumental communication, pay, promotional opportunity, and routinization. Three determinants do not appear to be important: integration, distributive justice, and professionalism. Age, length of service, and amount of time worked also appear to be important correlates. Variables which are important to the bivariate analysis, however, often turn out to be unimportant in the multivariate analysis. In fact, only with the multivariate analysis will it be possible to address the major questions of the relative importance of the variables and whether they operate in the manner indicated by the model.

Finally, when the means for the leavers and stayers were examined, all of the determinants except pay operated in the expected direction. In addition, the differences in means for the leavers and stayers were in the expected directions for age and length of service.

The inconsistent results for pay may be the consequence of combining the full-time nurses and the part-time nurses. The average pay for these two categories of nurses differs considerably, with the full-time nurses having an average pay of $10,298, while the part-time nurses receive an average of $5,422. There is also more diversity among the part-time nurses with respect to the number of hours worked. All the full-time nurses work a forty-hour week, whereas there is no set number of hours worked by the part-time nurses. When the leavers and stayers are examined, with amount of time worked controlled, the results for the full-time nurses are in accord with our expectations: the mean for the leavers is slightly lower ($10,208) than the mean for the stayers ($10,320). The results for the part-time nurses, however, depart from our expectations, since the leavers obtain a higher mean on pay ($5,766) than the stayers ($5,431).

The general impression at this point is that the zero-order results are mostly consistent with our model. It remains to be seen, however, whether the results are consistent with the model when statistical controls are used in the analysis.

NOTES

1. See Rosenberg (1968) for a discussion of suppressor variables.

CHAPTER 5
The Individual as the Unit of Analysis—The Entire Sample

The results of our multivariate analysis will be presented in the next three chapters. It was previously noted that two units of analysis are used, the individual and the immediate work group. When the individual is the unit, turnover is a dichotomous variable (each individual is either a "leaver" or a "stayer"), and the determinants have been measured for each nurse. When the nursing unit is used to analyze the data, turnover is a rate for each unit, and the pooled scores of the nurses who are members of the units are used to measure the determinants. This chapter and the following one present data which use the individual as the unit of analysis, whereas the seventh chapter presents data for nursing units. In this chapter the model is estimated for the entire sample of nurses, and in the following chapter it is estimated for four distinct categories of nurses.

RESULTS

Regression results for the entire sample of individual nurses are given in Table 5-1. Although turnover is the dependent variable in our research, it is customary in path analysis to refer also to the two intervening variables, intent to stay and job satisfaction, as "dependent variables." To conform to this custom, Table 5-1 presents several equations for each of the three dependent variables: job satisfaction, intent to stay, and turnover. Our focus in Table 5-1 is on the standardized partial regression coefficients (the "betas"), which may be directly compared with each other.

Job Satisfaction As the Dependent Variable

Seven variables are statistically significant when job satisfaction is regressed on all variables in the model except intent to stay and turnover (see Column 1): routinization, instrumental communication, promotional opportunity, participation, amount of time worked, kinship responsibility, and opportunity.[1] Four of these seven relationships are in agreement with expectations based on the model. Increased routinization was expected to result in reduced job satisfaction, and the results indicate that nurses whose jobs are very repetitive do express the greatest dissatisfaction with their work. Increased instrumental communication, promotional opportunity, and participation were expected to increase job satisfaction.

Table 5-1: Regression Results for Turnover, Intent to Stay, and Job Satisfaction As Dependent Variables for Total Sample

	Job Satisfaction				Intent to Stay				Turnover							
Independent Variables	b(1)	beta	b(2)	beta	b(3)	beta	b(4)	beta	b(5)	beta	b(6)	beta	b(7)	beta	b(8)	beta
Opportunity	-.11	-.08**	-.11	-.07*	-.09	-.12***	-.06	-.08 **	.03	.17 ***	.02	.16***	-.02	.12***	.02	.11***
Routinization	-.42	-.31***	-.43	-.31***	.03	.05	.03	.05	-.00	-.00	-.01	-.04	-.00	-.02	-.00	-.02
Participation	.13	.12***	-.14	-.12***	.03	.06	-.03	-.05	-.01	-.05	-.00	-.04	-.00	-.01	.00	.01
Instrumental Communication	.16	.21***	.16	.20***	.01	.02	-.01	-.01	-.00	-.05	-.00	-.03	-.00	-.02	-.00	-.01
Integration	.03	.04	.04	.06*	.01	.02	.01	.03	-.00	-.00	.00	.00	.00	.01	.00	.00
Pay[a]	.00	.04	.00	.04	.01	.09*	.00	.06	.00	.02	.00	.03	.00	.06	.00	.07
Distributive Justice	.03	.01	.04	.02	.03	.02	.03	.03	-.00	-.02	-.00	-.02	-.00	-.01	-.00	-.01
Promotional Opportunity	.11	.17***	.11	.16***	.02	.05	.02	.06 *	-.00	-.02	-.00	-.01	.00	.01	.00	.01
Professionalism	-.09	-.03	-.11	-.04	.04	.03	.03	.02	-.00	-.00	-.00	-.01	.00	.00	.00	.01
General Training	.25	.05	.24	.05	-.51	-.19***	-.36	-.13 ***	.07	.29 ***	.07	.13	.03	.06*	.03	.05
Kinship Responsibility	.24	.08*	.19	.06	.27	.17***	.17	.11 ***	-.02	-.07 *	-.02	-.06	-.00	-.00	.01	.02
Amount of Time Worked	-.92	-.11*	-.90	-.11*	.03	.01	.22	.05	-.06	-.07	-.07	-.08	-.07	-.08	-.08	-.09
Job Satisfaction					.13	.26***	.13	.26 ***			-.01	-.11 ***	-.00	-.01	-.00	-.01
Intent to Stay													-.07	-.37 ***	-.07	-.35 ***
Age			.05	.12***			.01	.06							-.00	-.05
Length of Service			-.21	-.07			.36	.26 ***							-.01	-.05
$R^2/\bar{R}^2$	.27	.26	.28	.27	.20	.19	.25	.24	.07	.06	.08	.07	.18	.17	.19	.18
N = 1,010 (Minimum pairwise N)																
N = 1,091 (Maximum pairwise N)																

[a] The unstandardized coefficients for pay are multiplied by 100.

* $p < .05$.

** $p < .01$.

*** $p < .001$.

The results indicate that when nurses are given information about their job, have the opportunity to get ahead occupationally in the hospitals, and participate in making job-related decisions, then their job satisfaction increases.

The significant effects for kinship responsibility and opportunity, while not expected on the basis of the model, are understandable. Kinship responsibility, it may be recalled, was expected to have an impact on turnover through intent to stay. Although the demographic literature, which suggested the kinship-responsibility-turnover proposition, indicated no mediating linkage between kinship responsibility and turnover, we developed a model which included intent to stay as a mediating variable. It is plausible, however, that kinship responsibility also has an impact on turnover through job satisfaction. The results in Column 1 are consistent with this possibility since strong ties to local kin—spouses and children in our research—produce increased job satisfaction.[2]

Opportunity is found to have a negative impact on job satisfaction. This means that the existence of alternative jobs outside the hospitals produces decreased job satisfaction among the nurses. Although this direct effect was not expected, such an impact makes sense. Environmental variables, such as opportunity, can and apparently do have an influence on the internal orientations of organizational members. What exists in the organization's environment influences the way its members view the work—in this case, satisfaction with their jobs.

It was previously noted that amount of time worked was used as a control variable because the sample consists of full-time and part-time nurses. Since the monetary incomes of these nurses are so different, without such a control the influence of pay might be obscured, if such an influence exists. The results indicate that the full-time nurses evidence less job satisfaction than the part-time nurses. These results were unexpected, and since there has been relatively little research on part-time employees, the literature does not provide us with a ready interpretation.

An examination of the magnitudes of the significant coefficients indicates that routinization is clearly the most important determinant of job satisfaction. Its beta coefficient is approximately 50 percent higher than the coefficient for instrumental communication, the second most important determinant. Routinization's coefficient is almost twice the size of the coefficient for promotional opportunity and two and a half times the size of the coefficient for participation, the third and fourth most important determinants. The coefficients for kinship responsibility and opportunity are about one-fourth the size of routinization's coefficient and are just barely statistically significant.

Intent to Stay As the Dependent Variable

When intent to stay is regressed on all determinants in the model (see Column 3), the following five variables are statistically significant: job satisfaction, general training, kinship responsibility, opportunity, and pay. The results for job satisfaction, general training, and kinship responsibility are in agreement with the model. As expected, the results indicate that nurses who like their jobs and who have local kin, such as spouses and children, are less likely to indicate that they will leave the hospitals than nurses who dislike their jobs and have fewer local kin. It was also expected that more general training would decrease intent to stay. Nurses with the most general training, those trained in colleges and universities (the baccalaureate nurses), are characterized by less intent to stay in the hospitals than nurses with the least general training, those trained in hospitals (the diploma nurses). It should be remembered that the nurses trained in junior colleges (the associate nurses) are located midway between the baccalaureate nurses and the diploma nurses on the measure of general training.

Even though the model does not hypothesize opportunity and pay as direct determinants of intent to stay, these observed effects are plausible. Most of the literature dealing with opportunity indicates that it has a direct impact on turnover; no intervening variables are specified. Our results suggest that nurses who have alternative jobs available outside the hospitals plan to leave and, as will soon be indicated, subsequently leave. Intent to stay is an intervening variable whereby the existence of alternative jobs is translated into turnover. The model also hypothesizes that the impact of pay on turnover is mediated by job satisfaction rather than by intent to stay. However, the regression results indicate that increased pay directly increases the intent to stay in the hospitals, that is, nurses who receive more pay indicate a greater intent to stay than nurses who receive less pay. Since pay is a major reward associated with work, it is plausible that it could have a direct impact on the nurses' intent to remain in the hospitals.

Job satisfaction is the most important determinant of intent to stay. The coefficient for job satisfaction is about half again as large as the coefficient for general training and kinship responsibility. Its net influence is twice the magnitude of the influence of opportunity and almost three times the size of the influence of pay.

Turnover As the Dependent Variable

Three determinants are statistically significant when turnover is regressed on all variables in the model (see Column 7): intent to stay, opportunity, and general training. The results for intent to stay and opportunity are in agreement with the model: the stronger the intent to stay, the less the turnover, and the greater the opportunity, the greater the turnover. Intent to stay, it may be recalled, is one dimension of commitment as defined in the important work by Porter and his colleagues (Mowday et al. 1979). The results are thus consistent with the claim that the more committed nurses are less likely to leave the hospitals.

The model does not indicate a direct path from general training to turnover, but rather suggests only that intent to stay mediates the general-training-turnover relationship. The previous results for intent to stay supported such a mediating role for intent to stay. The results now suggest that increased general training also directly influences turnover. Nurses with baccalaureate training (whose training is most general) are more likely to leave the hospitals than nurses with diploma training (whose training is most specific).

These data lead us to conclude that intent to stay is clearly the most important direct determinant of turnover. Its coefficient is slightly more than three times the size of opportunity's coefficient and nine times the size of the coefficient for general training.

Explained Variance

Table 5-1 also contains information about explained variance for each of the three dependent variables. The explained variances, respectively, for job satisfaction, intent to stay, and turnover are 26 percent, 19 percent, and 17 percent. Here and elsewhere, "explained variance" refers to "the adjusted R^2," which takes into account the sample size and the number of variables in the model. The adjusted R^2 is a conservative estimate of the explained variance. The model is most successful, using explained variance as the criterion, with respect to job satisfaction and is least successful with respect to turnover.

The Correlates: Age and Length of Service

Presentation of the results to this point has ignored age and length of service, two important and well-documented correlates of turnover. The earlier description of the model indicated that age and length of service would be used to assess the model by examining the explained variance with and without the use of these correlates. If the addition of these correlates to the model results in a significant increase in the explained variance, then we may conclude that the model has excluded determinants of turnover which are presently unknown but which are related to age and length of service. Since a great many variables change with an individual's increased age and length of service, use of these correlates constitutes an important check of the model.

Before presenting the results of adding age and length of service to the model, it is instructive to examine the zero-order correlation coefficients of age and length of service with the determinants in our model. In Chapter 3 we argued that exclusion of the correlates from the model is partly based on empirical assumptions about these zero-order coefficients. The zero-order coefficients to check these assumptions are contained in Table 5-2.

Table 5-2: Zero-Order Correlation Coefficients for the Determinants with Age and Length of Service

Variables	Age	Length of Service
Intent to Stay	.29	.36
Job Satisfaction	.12	.07
Opportunity	-.17	-.23
Routinization	.05	-.02
Participation	.03	.05
Instrumental Communication	.14	.16
Integration	-.18	-.01
Pay	-.11	-.11
Distributive Justice	-.02	.00
Promotional Opportunity	-.01	-.08
Professionalism	.03	.02
General Training	-.24	-.34
Kinship Responsibility	.35	.33

To simplify the presentation, only the statistically significant coefficients will be considered.[3] The results indicate that with increased age there is increased intent to stay, greater job satisfaction, decreased opportunity, better knowledge about the work, fewer close friends, less pay, less general training, and more kinship responsibility. Only the results for close friends and pay are contrary to expectations; we expected close friends and pay to increase with age.

The correlations indicate that with increased length of service there is increased intent to stay, greater job satisfaction, decreased opportunity, reduced pay, less general training, and more kinship responsibilities. Only the results for pay are contrary to expectations; we expected pay to increase with length of service.

In short, most of our empirical assumptions about the correlates are confirmed; they mostly vary in expected ways with the determinants.[4] We have argued that use of the determinants in the model makes it unnecessary also to use the correlates in the model. Our argument is that the determinants indicate what it is about the correlates that produce the relationships which are commonly found between the correlates and turnover.

The addition of age and length of service to the model results in an increase of .008 in the explained variance for job satisfaction, of .051 for intent to stay, and of .004 for turnover. Although the increase in explained variance for job satisfaction is very small, it is statistically significant, and as may be observed in Column 2 of Table 5-1, it is only age that has a significant influence. The R^2 increase for intent to stay is also significant, but it is length of service that is the important correlate here (see Column 4). The increase for turnover is not statistically significant, however (also see Column 8). What is most important is that the increase in the explained variance for intent to stay is relatively large, and we must conclude that one or more unknown variables, related primarily to length of service, probably are having an important impact on intent to stay.

The major results of the analysis can now be presented by means of a path diagram, which easily summarizes the data just presented (see Figure 5-1). The coefficients (path coefficients which equal betas) in the diagram are obtained by estimating the model again with all paths excluded which were not statistically significant. Exclusion of these paths results in path coefficients in the diagram slightly different from the betas in Table 5-1.

TOTAL EFFECTS

One of our objectives is to draw some inferences about the relative importance of the various determinants of turnover which have been identified as important in the literature. An examination of the net effects (Table 5-1, Column7) is informative but incomplete for this purpose. Because the turnover model includes two intervening variables, it is possible to identify the total causal effect of each variable. In particular, we can identify three types of variables: (1) those having only direct effects (intent to stay); (2) those having both direct and indirect effects opportunity, kinship responsibility, and general training); and (3) those having only indirect effects (all the other determinants).

By means of path-analytic techniques, it is possible to add the direct and indirect effects for opportunity and general training to obtain an indication of their total effects on turnover. The total effects of the remaining eight determinants will be equal to either their direct or their indirect effects. Examination of these total effects for the thirteen determinants (see Table 5-3) shows the rank order to be as follows: intent to stay (-.37), opportunity (.16), general training (.13), job satisfaction (-.10), kinship responsibility (-.07), pay (-.04), routinization (.03), instrumental communication (-.02), promotional opportunity (-.02), and participation (-.01). Integration, distributive justice, and professionalism have no total effect.

Although these total effects have allowed us to reach our objective of rank-ordering the determinants, two cautionary notes are pertinent. First, one must not view the results too rigidly. Slight differences in total effects—one or two points—between determinants should not be viewed as meaningful. The ranking which we discuss, in short, should be viewed as a relatively crude ordering of the determinants. Second, we view total effects of .05 or less as not substantially meaningful. This criterion is,

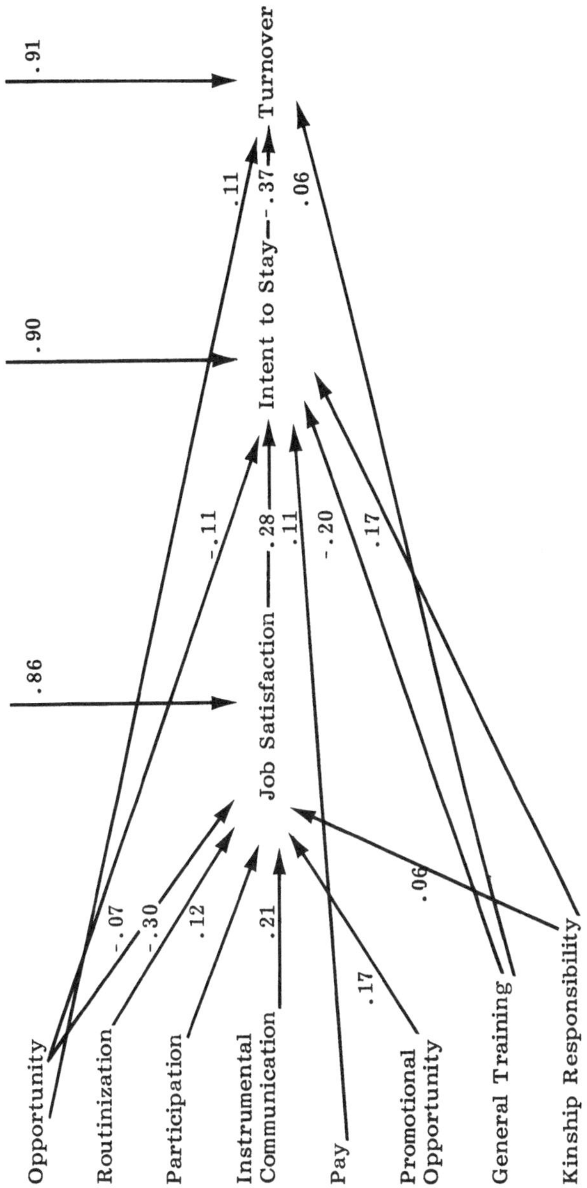

Figure 5-1: Results of Estimation of Causal Model for Entire Sample of Nurses

Table 5-3: Direct, Indirect, and Total Effects for the Whole Sample

Variables	Direct Effects	Indirect Effects Via: Job Satisfaction	Intent to Stay	Job Satisfaction and Intent to Stay	Total Effects
Intent to Stay	-.37	ns	--	--	-.37
Job Satisfaction	ns[a]	--	-.10	--	-.10
Opportunity	.11	ns	.04	.01	.16
Routinization	ns	ns	ns	.03	.03
Participation	ns	ns	ns	-.01	-.01
Instrumental Communication	ns	ns	ns	-.02	-.02
Integration	ns	ns	ns	ns	ns
Pay	ns	ns	-.04	ns	-.04
Distributive Justice	ns	ns	ns	ns	ns
Promotional Opportunity	ns	ns	ns	-.02	-.02
Professionalism	ns	ns	ns	ns	ns
General Training	.06	ns	.07	ns	.13
Kinship Responsibility	ns	ns	-.06	-.01	-.07
Amount of Time Worked	ns	ns	ns	.01	.01

[a]Not statistically significant.

of course, an arbitrary dividing point, but it does keep us from over-interpreting small effects. The determinants will be discussed (those with total effects greater than .05, that is) by order of magnitude, beginning with the largest, following some comments on the intervening variables and the causal ordering of the variables in our model.

THE ROLE OF INTERVENING VARIABLES

As already discussed, the examination of direct effects is only part of the information available from a path model and, by itself, can sometimes be misleading. Also, as already mentioned, one of the major arguments appearing in the recent turnover literature is that the organizational characteristics produce varying levels of satisfaction, which, in turn, influence the person's commitment to the organization, which, in turn, is the major direct determinant of turnover. In short, there are expected indirect effects which must be examined.

An overall estimate of indirect effects may be obtained by computing various "sheaf coefficients" for the exogenous determinants (all determinants except job satisfaction and intent to stay) as a block of variables. As described by Heise (1972), the sheaf coefficient is comparable to a path coefficient, but is unique because it represents the combined influence of a set of several variables. The total causal influence of the exogenous determinants is .26 and is obtained by computing the sheaf coefficient for turnover regressed only on these variables. The total net (unmediated) effects of these determinants is .15, which is the sheaf coefficient after controlling for job satisfaction and intent to stay. The total net effect, controlling only for job satisfaction, is .25. From this information we may say that 3.8 percent ($1 - \frac{.25}{.26}$) of the total causal influence of the determinants operates through job satisfaction, 38.5 percent ($\frac{.25-.15}{.26}$) operates through intent to stay, while 57.7 percent ($\frac{.15}{.26}$) of the total effect of the determinants is direct (unmediated by job satisfaction, intent to stay, or both). Thus, the importance of intent to stay as an intervening variable is demonstrated.

The separate indirect effects of particular determinants (rather than as a block) through satisfaction and intent may be assessed by comparing the standardized coefficients in the reduced form model (Column 5, where satisfaction and intent are removed) with the same coefficients in the model with these two variables included (Columns 6 and 7). For example, when only satisfaction is added, the influence of general training is not altered (compare Columns 5 and 6). However, when intent to stay is then added (Column 7), the coefficient is reduced from .13 to .06, indicating that over half of the total causal effect of this variable is mediated by intent to stay.

The importance of intent to stay in the model is not just its significance as an intervening variable, however. First, it contributes significantly to the explained variation in turnover. As may be seen by comparing Column 6 with Column 7 in Table 5-1, its net contribution is 10 percent. Second, excluding intent to stay from the model results in concluding that job satisfaction is more important than it actually is (compare the coefficient for satisfaction in the same two equations).

A NOTE ON CAUSAL ORDERING

Our review of the turnover literature convinced us that job satisfaction should be represented as being causally prior to intent to stay. However, the hypothesis that job satisfaction influences intent to stay rather than vice versa cannot be directly tested with our data because both variables are measured at the same point in time. LISREL (Jöreskog and Sorböm 1978), however, which utilizes the additional statistical information made available when there are multiple indicators of constructs, can be used to estimate the magnitude of reciprocal effects between variables, thereby providing some empirical data about causal ordering. Using it to estimate such effects between job satisfaction and intent to stay, we find the path from intent to stay to job satisfaction (the opposite of what we hypothesized) to be .12, a statistically nonsignificant value; the path from job satisfaction to intent to stay (the hypothesized effect) is a statistically significant value of .31. Although this cannot be interpreted as proof of the causal-ordering assumption of the model, it certainly is consistent with it. In addition, if, as is commonly done in causal analysis, nonsignificant paths are eliminated and the model is then reestimated, the results are consistent with our causal model, that is, one with the path going from job satisfaction to intent to stay. The appendix at the end of the chapter provides additional information on the LISREL analysis.

DISCUSSION

Intent to stay is clearly the most important determinant of turnover. Its total effects are more than twice the size of the total effects for the second most important determinant, opportunity, and its importance as an intervening variable is clearly indicated. Research on the determinants of turnover has generally ignored intent to stay in favor of job satisfaction. Since intent to stay is one dimension of commitment, the results support the contention of Porter and his colleagues (Mowday et al. 1979) that commitment is a more important determinant of turnover than job satisfaction. The relative importance accorded intent to stay is one of the most significant results of our research. No longer can this variable be excluded from research on the determinants of turnover.

Opportunity is the second most important determinant of turnover. Economists who stress this variable are correct: alternative jobs in the environment do play a major role in producing turnover. What is especially interesting in the results is the relative importance of pay and opportunity. There is a very substantial body of literature supporting these two determinants, and it has been difficult to ascertain their relative importance because the economists who mostly deal with these variables do not include in their models determinants emphasized by sociologists and social psychologists. The relative importance of pay and opportunity must be examined with all other determinants controlled, and our multivariate analysis provides this type of data. Our results indicate that opportunity is a more important determinant than pay; the coefficient for opportunity is twice the size of the coefficient for pay. March and Simon, as may be recalled, argued (1958) that opportunity is the most important determinant of turnover. Although this role, as just indicated, goes to intent to stay rather than to opportunity, March and Simon's position is given some support.

Economists who emphasize opportunity stress its direct impact on turnover, and our results support this view of opportunity because we find a direct effect of .11 (Table 5-3). However, our results (Table 5-3) also indicate that opportunity has indirect effects on turnover of .05 (.04 through intent to stay and .01 through job satisfaction and intent to stay). Although the direct effects are more than twice the indirect effects, thus supporting the emphasis of economists, the indirect effects exist and must not be ignored. Our results about opportunity's indirect effects should be viewed as supplementing the work of economists and as supportive of the previous work of Bluedorn (1976) and Martin (1977). As far as we know, Bluedorn is the first researcher to suggest that opportunity's impact on turnover might be indirect. His data, and later that of Martin, supports this suggestion. Unlike Bluedorn and Martin, however, we stress both the direct and indirect effects of opportunity.

We do not intend to leave the impression that economists (and now we) are the only behavioral scientists who examine the impact of environmental variables on the organization and its members. Organizational scholars have traditionally neglected environmental variables as determinants, focusing instead on other organizational properties as producers of their dependent variables. Organizational effectiveness, for instance, will often be explained by the nature of the work, power, and control structures of organizations— thus completely ignoring environmental variables, such as abundance of resources. Recently, however, a growing number of organizational scholars have begun to emphasize the importance of environmental variables as determinants of organizational properties. The stimulating work of Aldrich (1979) and Pfeffer and Salancik (1978) illustrates different aspects of the growing emphasis on the importance of environmental determinants of organizational properties. Our emphasis on opportunity as a determinant of turnover should be viewed as part of the attempt to stress the importance of environmental variables.

General training is the third-ranking determinant; its total effects are almost 90 percent of the size of those for opportunity. Becker's insight (1962, 1964) on this matter is correct: training which improves the productivity of individuals in diverse organizations promotes turnover more than training specific to an organization. In our sample this means that baccalaureate training results in greater turnover than diploma training.

The importance accorded general training is somewhat surprising. It has little empirical support in the literature and its measurement in our research is crude. The results about general training mean that two of the three most important determinants are those emphasized by economists. Sociologists and social psychologists have been seriously remiss in ignoring these two determinants; they should be included in all models of turnover. It might also be noted, however, that most economists have also ignored general training in their research, since the only empirical support we could find for the general-training-turnover proposition is the work by Parsons (1972).

Although intent to stay is a more important determinant than job satisfaction, the results do indicate job satisfaction to be important. Only opportunity and general training are more important than job satisfaction. Its total effects are almost 70 percent those of opportunity and almost 80 percent those of general training. So even though we must downplay the importance of job satisfaction when compared to the three determinants just discussed, we cannot dismiss the claim of the many scholars who have assigned an important role to job satisfaction. What is significant about our research is that we suggest, and our results support, that job satisfaction has an indirect influence through intent to stay: increases in job satisfaction produce greater intent to stay, which, in turn, result in less turnover.[6] If intent to stay can be viewed as a dimension of commitment, and this is appropriate if the Porter view of commitment is accepted, then our results are in agreement with the work of Mobley (1977) and Brief (Brief and Aldag 1977), who explicitly assigned a mediating role to commitment. Future research on the determinants of turnover must include job satisfaction and commitment in the models to be tested.

Kinship responsibility is the fifth most important determinant. Local kin, especially spouse and children, decrease the likelihood of turnover. The importance accorded kinship responsibility is surprising in view of the fact that we borrowed it from the demography literature on migration and we did not measure it as well as we would have liked.

Our results for kinship responsibility are relevant to the classic Porter and Steers review (1973, pp. 166-167) which cites the significance of "family responsibility" as a determinant of turnover. They state that increased family responsibility produces more turnover for women, whereas the results for men are mixed. Seldom is any mention of the family to be found in the turnover literature; Porter and Steers thus perform a valuable service in reminding us of an easily overlooked variable.[7] What is really surprising, however, is that our results do not support the Porter and Steers conclusion, since we find that increased kinship responsibility decreases turnover in our sample of female nurses.

The results for kinship responsibility should also be viewed in a larger context. Organizational research generally ignores kinship variables, but when such variables are mentioned, the focus is usually on the impact of the organization on the kinship systems. A favorite topic in this connection is how the rotation of the executive within the organization, which commonly involves migration, disrupts the executive's family (Whyte 1956). When it is allowed that kinship variables might have an impact on organizations, the impact suggested is always negative. The Porter and Steers review (1973) is illustrative of such a negative impact: family responsibilities increase turnover for women. And increased turnover, as the first chapter indicated, threatens effectiveness and decreases productivity. A common point made when examining the impact of the kinship system on the organization is the threat posed by the family to the organization's customary emphasis on merit. Organizations have generally sought to exclude family considerations (nepotism rules are an example) from their operations.[8]

Our data indicate the positive impact of a kinship variable on the organization: kinship responsibilities decrease turnover. These results must naturally be replicated elsewhere, and with improved measurement. If the results hold, we will have learned that a commonly neglected variable, the existence of local kin, has a seldom-suggested positive impact on organizations, the reduction of its turnover.

Kinship responsibility, finally, should be related to the preceding discussion of opportunity as an environmental variable. We also intend kinship responsibility to be another environmental variable. Our research primarily emphasizes the spouse and children as the source of kinship responsibility (Appendix B at the end of the book), and these individuals are, of course, nearly always located in the organization's environment. The measurement of ties to additional relatives should also be added in future research on this determinant, such as the parents and siblings of the spouses. These parents and siblings are also located outside the organization and are thus part of its environment. With better measurement, kinship responsibility may be found to be an even more important environmental variable.

The remaining eight determinants have total effects of less than .05 and are thus considered not substantively significant. Each of these determinants, however, requires a brief discussion.

Two comments about pay are pertinent. First, the amount of literature supporting pay as a determinant is much more extensive than the literature supporting general training and kinship responsibility—yet the latter two determinants have total effects considerably larger than pay. The total effects for general training and kinship responsibility are, respectively, more than three times and almost twice the total effects for pay. Increased pay results in decreased turnover, but specific training and greater kinship responsibility result in even greater reductions in turnover. This result is unexpected but plausible and could only have been obtained by means of multivariate analysis. The value of examining the impact of the determinants on turnover with all other major determinants controlled is again demonstrated. Future research which seeks to explain variations in turnover must move away from an emphasis on bivariate relationships (zero-order relationships) toward an emphasis on multivariate analysis.

These results about pay—and this is the second comment—are relevant to the current discussion about the significance of pay for professional employees. Some scholars (Lyons 1968; McGee 1971; National Opinion Research Center 1972) deemphasize the importance of pay for professional employees, whereas others (Blau 1974) place relatively more stress on the motive power of pay for professional employees. The results of our research support the scholars who deemphasize the value of pay for professional employees. Nurses are professional employees and pay is less important than intent to stay, opportunity, general training, job satisfaction, and kinship responsibility. Our results, however, do not indicate that pay is totally unimportant for professional employees. Although less than .05, the total effects for pay are larger than the total effects for the remaining seven determinants. Thus, for the nurses in our sample, pay, although not of much importance, is of some significance.

One final note of caution should be mentioned regarding the weak effect of pay. Pay may have been strongly stressed in the literature, at least in part, because most of the previous research has been performed on full-time workers. Since full-time workers are typically primary wage-earners, it could be expected that pay would be more important for this type of worker. As more nurses become primary wage earners—through, for instance, careers without marriage and the establishment of single-parent families—it is expected that pay will become more important. Although the data are not clear, it does seem that proportionately more nurses are becoming primary wage-earners. Future research may indicate that pay is more important for nurses than it now seems.

We find it interesting that routinization, promotional opportunity, distributive justice, and professionalism are classified together with instrumental communication, participation, and integration as having essentially zero total effects. The volume of literature supporting the first four determinants is much smaller than the quantity of data supporting the last three determinants. Only pay and opportunity are supported by more data than instrumental communication, participation, and integration. Two respected scholars, Van der Merwe and Miller, even suggest (1970, p.24) that integration is the most important of the determinants. Yet when the seven determinants are included in the same model, their effects are essentially zero. This is the type of result which could only have been obtained by multivariate analysis and is one of the major findings of our research.

As we can illustrate with integration, distributive justice, and professionalism, it is not yet time to discard these seven determinants from future research in this area. It is possible that *integration* did not turn out to be important because its measurement stresses close friends in the work organization rather than in the immediate work group (Appendix B). It is conceivable that what is really significant for turnover is the support of close friends in the immediate work group. This possibility should be checked before integration is discarded. Although our results support Mobley's (Mobley et al. 1979b, p. 503) review (he does not find a strong relationship between "peer group relations"—our "integration"—and turnover), Van der Merwe and Miller may yet turn out to be correct, or not so totally wrong.

It may be that the measurement of *distributive justice* is too narrow. The questionnaire items focus on the relationship between effort expended and pay (Appendix B). And pay is, of course, but one type of organizational reward. The allocation of recognition and physical facilities are, for example, organizational rewards excluded by the questionnaire's focus on pay. Although we find no empirical support for distributive justice, the support in the literature is fairly substantial and the concept should not be discarded until its measurement is improved.

It is conceivable that *professionalism* is not especially important because our sample of nurses was too heavily concentrated at the low end of the continuum of scores. The index of professionalism extends from one to twelve, but almost two-thirds (65.7) of the nurses are in the lowest category and almost 80 percent (77.6) of the nurses are in the lowest two categories. With greater dispersion of scores, professionalism may turn out to be of greater significance. Professionalism should not be excluded as a possible determinant until it is checked with a sample whose dispersion of scores is wider or until a more appropriate measure is found.

We have included a large number of determinants in our model, and this is contrary to the classic scientific preference for parsimony. However, our model is complex because the previous studies have not included all the major determinants in their models. We would like to eliminate the eight determinants whose total effects are basically zero. As just indicated, however, we can think of obvious reasons why integration, distributive justice, and professionalism should not yet be discarded. Perhaps equally obvious reasons exist for not yet discarding *routinization*, *participation*, instrumental communication, pay, and promotional opportunity. The point we wish to make is that these eight determinants should not be discarded until the suggested changes are made and the model is tested under different conditions. It will take some time before the model can be considerably simplified.

The work of economists and noneconomists has been often commented on during this discussion. It should be apparent that future research should include economic and noneconomic determinants in the models to be estimated. Opportunity, general training, and pay—determinants commonly stressed by economists—must be included in future research, as must intent to stay (but measured more generally as commitment), job satisfaction, kinship responsibility, routinization, participation, instrumental communication, integration, distributive justice, promotional opportunity, and professionalism—determinants commonly stressed by sociologists and social psychologists. Future tests of the model will probably indicate that both economic and noneconomic determinants are important. Choices will probably not have to be made in either/or terms.

One final comment about environmental variables is required. We have indicated that we view opportunity and kinship responsibility to be environmental determinants of turnover and thus to be in accord with the growing emphasis on the importance of this type of determinant. Most of our determinants, however, are the ones emphasized by traditional scholars. As it does not seem necessary for us to choose between economic or noneconomic determinants, so it does not seem necessary for us to select either environmental or organizational determinants of turnover. Both types of determinants appear to be important. Only future research will indicate the extent to which our traditional determinants are produced by the environment, but we anticipate finding that some variation continues to be produced by the organization. We prefer a moderate position between extreme neglect of the environment and an emphasis which explains all organizational variation by environmental determinants.

Explained Variance

The discussion to this point has exclusively focused on the relative importance of the variables producing variations in turnover. Providing such an ordering was one of the major purposes of our research. However, this research is also concerned with explaining as much as possible of the variation in turnover. There is little point in ordering a set of variables which have no explanatory power!

The explained variance of the model is 17 percent. As previously indicated, the reference, here as elsewhere, is to the adjusted R^2. This explained variance is less than the 23 percent cited in Mobley's recent review (Mobley et al. 1979b, pp. 510-512). We are disappointed by the size of our explained variance, since our model included all major determinants of turnover we could identify.

There are at least four possible reasons for our relatively low explained variance[9]. First, we may have excluded significant determinants. This issue was briefly discussed when the model was described. While this is a possiblity, we believe that our explained variance will not be significantly increased by the addition of more determinants. Our review of the turnover literature encompasses the research of hundreds of scholars working over a period of approximately 70 years, and it is unlikely that too much has been missed by these scholars. Our next project will, however, add several excluded variables to test for this possibility—to the chagrin, we are sure, of those who think we have already included far too many determinants! These variables will be identified in the concluding chapter. Such variables might be expected to increase our explained variance by only a few percentage points, however.

Second, our explained variance may be relatively low because of inadequate measurement. We are much more hopeful about increasing the explained variance by improvements in measurement. Needed improvements in measurement have been repeatedly mentioned in the preceding discussion, and the concluding chapter will draw together all of these measurement suggestions, plus a few others. However, our measurement is, on the whole, adequate, and dramatic improvements, such as doubling the explained variance, should not be expected from this change.

Third, our explained variance undoubtedly is low because of the long length of time between administration of the questionnaires and collection of the turnover data. The questionnaires, it may be recalled, were administered to the nurses in August 1976, and all of the determinants were measured by the questionnaire data. Approximately fourteen months later, in October 1977, the turnover data were collected from the seven hospitals. With the turnover data, the sample of nurses was divided into leavers and stayers. The data collected in August 1976 were thus used to explain variations in leaving and staying in October 1977.

It is likely that important changes occurred in the situations of the nurses during the fourteen-month period between data collection for the independent and dependent variables. Many of the nurses, for instance, probably received pay raises, since the fourteen months were an inflationary period in the United States. A few of the nurses also likely received promotions during this period of time, and if the promoted nurses continued to be employed by the hospitals, which is usually the case, they were counted as stayers. Some nurses also probably developed close friendships with other nurses, whereas other close friendships among some nurses dissolved. Finally, changes could also have occurred as the result of transfers between units within the hospitals or because of changes in supervisors.

It is likely that these changes also decreased our explained variance. Price's previously mentioned pilot study (Price and Bluedorn 1979) is instructive in this connection.[10] In his study, questionnaires were first administered to the nurses in February 1974, and turnover data were collected twelve months later, in February 1975. A second questionnaire was also administered in February 1975, and a second set of turnover data collected in February 1976. When the timespan is twelve months—when the differences between leavers and stayers in February 1975 are explained by data collected in February 1974—the explained variance is 23 percent. When the timespan is increased to twenty-four months—when the difference between leavers and stayers in February 1976 is explained by data collected in February 1974—the explained variance declines to 14 percent. The longer the span of time between data collection for the independent and dependent variables, the lower the explained variance.

Future research should not allow fourteen months to lapse between data collection for the independent and dependent variables. The concluding chapter will indicate how to obtain a large turnover rate in a shorter period of time, such as six months, between data collection for the independent and dependent variables. We believe that our explained variance can be considerably increased by shortening our lapsed time from fourteen to six months.

We should make one final comment about the long timespan. Although this long timespan probably decreased our explained variance, our confidence in the substantive results which we obtained is strengthened. Determinants which are still statistically significant after fourteen months are powerful determinants!

Fourth, only women (most of whom were married) were included in this study. Even with the current ideological and legal support for women's rights, the cultural norm still exists, which prescribes that the wife leave her job when the husband finds employment in another community. Our model does not include any variable which directly taps this contingency. Thus, the explained variance is smaller because of this.

Our 17 percent explained variance is, admittedly, discouraging, especially given our comprehensive model. We believe, however, that the explained variance can be significantly increased by the addition of a few more determinants to the model; by a series of substantial measurement improvements, including, most important, taking family contingencies more into account; and by considerably shortening the time span from fourteen to six months between data collection for the independent and dependent variables.

This concludes the presentation of the results for the entire sample of nurses at the individual level of analysis. The second step in presenting the results, still at the individual level of analysis, is to estimate the model for different categories of nurses. Results for this type of analysis are presented in the following chapter.

NOTES

1. An F test with 1 and n-k-1 degrees of freedom is used to assess statistical significance. (n = number of cases and k = number of independent variables in the equation.)

2. We also have an evaluative dimension of kinship responsibility. (See Appendix B.)

3. Coefficients greater than $|\pm .06|$ are statistically significant at the 5 percent level.

4. The unexpected results for pay and integration are probably due to the inclusion of full-time and part-time nurses in our sample. Our expectations about the relationships between the correlates (age and length of service) and the determinants are based on data derived from the study of full-time employees. We have no clear expectations for the relationships between the correlates and the determinants for part-time employees.

5. There is, of course, also the possibility that improved measurement of our determinants will increase our ability to explain variance in intent to stay.

6. The material in Appendix 5-1 is pertinent at this point.

7. Tainio (1977) also has data relevant to our material about kinship responsibility.

8. Max Weber's material on bureaucracy is significant here. See Albrow (1970) for an excellent general discussion of bureaucracy.

9. Our explained variance, however, is not low compared to other studies of nursing turnover. See, for example, the work of Sloan (1975; 1978; 135-165). We should also note that nonlinearity does not explain our low explained variance. See our discussion of the assumptions of multiple regression and path analysis in Chapter 3.

10. The statistics which we report in this paragraph are not included in the published version of the pilot study.

APPENDIX 5-1

LISREL is a general statistical model for the analysis of Linear Structural Relationships among variables. Jöreskog (1973) introduced the technique, which has undergone several revisions, with LISREL IV currently being the preferred computer program (Jöreskog and Sorböm 1978). The technique uses maximum-likelihood estimation procedures to fit and test various models of linear structural relationships among variables. The procedure allows for including both observed (measured) variables and unobserved (latent) constructs in the same model. The latent variables may have one or more measures, which can be fallible, that is, unreliable indicators. The unreliability of these measures is taken into account in obtaining estimates of the relationships among the latent variables. Standard errors of all estimates are produced, thus allowing for assessing statistical significance.

When there exist multiple indicators of the latent constructs which make the equations identified, it is possible to estimate the reciprocal effects between latent variables. This is precisely what we have done in an attempt to provide support for the causal ordering we assume between job satisfaction and intent to stay.

The LISREL model we estimated is like that depicted in Figure 2-1 except for the following differences. First, reciprocal paths between job satisfaction and intent to stay are included. Second, the seven indicators of job satisfaction and the two indicators of intent to stay are included in the model (they are used to form indexes in the other analysis we report), thus providing enough additional information for the technique to estimate the reciprocal relationships between the two latent constructs, job satisfaction and intent to stay. We constrained the other paths in the model to correspond to those in Figure 2-1 and assumed uncorrelated error variances for the indicators of job satisfaction and intent to stay. The correlation matrix was analyzed and the standardized solution used. The correlation between the residuals for satisfaction and intent to stay is -.08, and the LISREL path estimate from job satisfaction to turnover is a nonsignificant .023, whereas the path from intent to stay to turnover is -.424. This represents still more evidence that intent to stay is the more important determinant of the two. The test for goodness of fit produces a chi square value of 380 with 130 degrees of freedom. We must remind the reader, however, that the robustness of LISREL under violation of the assumption of a continuous dependent variable is not well understood (Stapleton 1977).

CHAPTER 6
The Individual as the Unit of Analysis—The Four Categories

Our analysis thus far has rested on the assumption that the turnover of nonsupervisory registered nurses may be explained by a single causal model of how the determinants operate to produce the turnover. We are, however, quite aware that there may exist no such single model, but instead there may exist several models, each appropriate for nurses with different characteristics. It is our objective in this chapter to determine if the model described in the preceding chapter is appropriate for particular categories of nurses.

IDENTIFYING RELEVANT CATEGORIES-

Estimating the causal model for differing categories of nurses requires selection of relevant categories, that is, theoretically as well as empirically distinct categories. Unfortunately, no assistance is available from the literature to make this selection because most researchers have assumed a single model is appropriate for all populations.[1] Initially, therefore, we must select our categories using pragmatic and intuitive criteria.

Amount of time worked would seem to be one of the most important differentiating characteristics of nurses. The fieldwork connected with this research, plus Price's previous fieldwork (Price and Bluedorn 1979) on a similar hospital, has indicated a belief among hospital administrators that full-time nurses are very different from part-time nurses. The model may consequently be different, in some important respects, for the full-time nurses and the part-time nurses. It is also wise to treat these two categories of nurses differently to obtain a more refined statistical control for pay. Full-time and part-time nurses differ considerably in the pay they receive, and this difference is not totally captured by the controls introduced by regression analysis.

The model may also work differently for nurses who differ by length of service and age. Farrell's research (1978) on the determinants of job satisfaction finds that the variables which influence job satisfaction vary by amount of experience in the labor force. Since job satisfaction is an important determinant of turnover, Farrell's results are relevant to our research.[2] Length of service, while not equivalent to labor-force experience, can be expected to operate similarly.[3] Use of length of service as a variable for categorizing nurses is also supported by its well-documented negative relationship with turnover (Price 1977, pp. 26-28): organizational employees with short lengths of service usually have higher rates of turnover than employees with long length's of service. If the model is estimated for nurses categorized by length of service, then it also seems appropriate to consider differences by age. Like length of service, there is substantial empirical support (Price 1977, pp. 28-29) for the negative relationship of age and turnover. Length of service and age thus seem to be two additional variables useful in distinguishing the nurses.

As described in Chapter 3, we assess whether these pragmatically and intuitively derived variables used for categorizing produce empirically distinct groups of nurses by testing for whether the variables in the model interact with these three in their influence on the dependent variables. To do this, interaction terms were entered into the regression equation for amount of time worked, length of service, and age. The appendix at the end of this chapter describes how these interaction tests were conducted. When job satisfaction is the dependent variable, only amount-of-time-worked interactions are significant. When intent to stay is viewed as the dependent variable, significant interactions are found for amount-of-time-worked and age, but not for length of service. When turnover is viewed as the dependent variable, significant interactions are found for age and length-of-service interactions, but not for amount of time worked. In sum, statistically significant interactions exist in various forms with these three correlates. This means a model should be estimated separately for various categories of nurses defined by combinations of these three correlates. It will then be possible to determine if these differences can be given a meaningful substantive interpretation.

The sample, however, is only large enough to subdivide by combinations of two correlates. We argue that amount of time worked must be retained because of the widespread belief that full-time nurses and part-time nurses are different and by the necessity of providing an unambiguous check on the key pay variable. Of the other two, age was selected instead of length of service because the categories of nurses obtained by using age had more clearly differentiated amounts of explained variance for the dependent variables (job satisfaction, intent to stay, and turnover) and because the practical implications associated with age are clearer. Cross-classification by amount of time worked and age, each divided into two categories, yields four categories of nurses: full-time under thirty (N = 434), full-time thirty and over (N = 184), part-time under thirty (N = 161), and part-time thirty and over (N = 218). The means and standard deviations for the variables for each of these four categories are contained in Table 6-1.

By comparing the means for turnover, we see clearly that it is the younger nurses who more often leave the hospital. Likewise, it is the younger nurses who are least likely to indicate an intent to stay. Not all of these differences are consistent with expectations or "common sense," however. For example, it is the full-time nurses who are more often placed in the most routine jobs. Also, although we would expect the full-time workers to participate more than the part-time workers in the decision making relevant to their jobs, the means do not allow us to conclude this. In sum, we caution against judging how these categories are different on the basis of these simple descriptive data.

We are mainly concerned with whether the model estimated in Figure 5-1 of the preceding chapter accurately depicts how the various determinants operate to produce turnover for the four categories of nurses we have identified. To do this we must examine the regression coefficients, as was done in the preceding chapter. However, as has been described and discussed numerous times (Blalock 1967; Kim and Mueller 1976), comparisons of causal models across different populations must be based on

Table 6-1: Variable Means and Standard Deviations for Four Categories of Nurses

Variables	Full-time Under Thirty X	Full-time Under Thirty SD	Full-time Thirty and Over X	Full-time Thirty and Over SD	Part-time Under Thirty X	Part-time Under Thirty SD	Part-time Thirty and Over X	Part-time Thirty and Over SD
Turnover	.24	.43	.08	.28	.30	.46	.11	.32
Intent to Stay	5.84	1.94	7.35	1.94	6.05	2.07	6.88	1.92
Job Satisfaction	27.66	3.92	28.45	4.72	28.34	3.71	29.25	3.60
Opportunity	11.81	2.59	10.94	2.78	11.46	2.68	10.95	2.73
Routinization	11.96	2.86	12.19	3.05	11.85	2.98	11.74	2.91
Participation	13.82	3.35	14.00	3.86	13.81	3.17	13.94	3.53
Instrumental Communication	25.95	4.91	27.53	5.33	25.71	4.90	26.72	4.84
Integration	9.93	5.35	7.67	5.02	8.17	4.99	6.71	4.85
Pay	$10,157	$1,526	$10,644	$1,546	$5,849	$2,404	$5,113	$2,273
Distributive Justice	6.95	1.58	6.79	1.74	7.24	1.57	7.15	1.65
Promotional Opportunity	21.76	5.78	21.07	6.45	21.29	5.78	22.11	6.41
Professionalism	1.82	1.37	2.08	1.53	1.60	1.29	1.61	1.17
General Training	1.66	.85	1.26	.61	1.47	.73	1.19	.54
Kinship Responsibility	4.03	1.32	5.32	1.04	5.52	1.03	5.68	.76
Age	23.74	2.38	44.32	8.76	25.45	2.32	40.26	8.39
Length of Service	2.38	.93	4.05	1.20	2.77	.98	3.90	1.22

the examination of the unstandardized coefficients (the b's) rather than on the standardized coefficients (the betas).

Our strategy will be, first, to identify in what ways the four categories of nurses are similar and, second, to identify how they are different. Given the large number of variables in the model, however, such comparisons can end up being very detailed and often confusing. As discussed in the appendix at the end of this chapter, it is impossible to conduct a statistical-significance test for whether the influence of each and every variable differs across the four categories of nurses. This unavailability of systematic testing procedures can lead to the application of rather arbitrary criteria in deciding where the similarities and differences lie. To avoid this, we have adopted the following convention: we will say that the influence of a determinant is similar if it is statistically significant for at least three of the four categories of nurses.[4] (By definition, then, differences will be said to exist if this statistical-significance criterion is not met.) There will, of course, be situations in which this criterion is met but the statistically significant coefficients differ substantially in magnitude, that is, where there actually are differences. In such instances, we will apply the general rule of thumb that for differences to be considered meaningful, a coefficient must be approximately twice as large as the others in the comparison.

The results for the regression analysis for each of the four categories of nurses are contained in Tables 6-2 through 6-5. The same format as used for the tables in the preceding chapter is used here. The complete correlation matrices for these four categories are in Appendix C at the end of the book.

SIMILARITIES AMONG THE NURSES

When job satisfaction is viewed as the dependent variable (see Column 1 of the tables), four determinants are statistically significant for at least three categories of nurses: routinization, participation, instrumental communication, and promotional opportunity. The influence of these determinants is in accordance with the causal model. Increases in routinization decrease job satisfaction, whereas increases in participation, instrumental communication, and promotional opportunity produce greater job satisfaction.

When intent to stay is the dependent variable (see Column 3), job satisfaction is the only determinant which is generally important, and as predicted by the model, increased job satisfaction results in greater intent to remain in the hospitals.

For turnover (see Column 7), only one determinant, intent to stay, is important for all categories of nurses. This result, as predicted by the model, shows that nurses indicating the strongest intent to stay are the least likely to leave the hospital.

To summarize, we have found that most nurses, regardless of age and amount of time worked, are similar in that six determinants operate to influence directly or indirectly the probability of their turnover. Greater variety in work, greater participation in work-related decisions, greater communication about work, and greater opportunity to advance in the hospital—all operate to increase job satisfaction. Higher job satisfaction, then, operates to increase intent to stay, which, in turn, operates to reduce the likelihood of turnover. Since we view intent to stay as a dimension of commitment, the results support the idea that increased commitment to the hospital reduces turnover.

DIFFERENCES AMONG CATEGORIES OF NURSES

There are four types of differences which we observe to exist across these four categories of nurses. First, a determinant is statistically significant and its influence is in the expected direction (that is, positive if expected to be positive), but these two conditions do not hold for all four categories of nurses. (This situation necessarily means that for some of the categories the expected effect is not observed.) Second, the variable is significant for only one or two categories, but it is not expected to be significant for any. Third, the influence of a determinant is significant for one or two categories, but the direction of the influence is opposite of what is expected. Fourth, the determinant is significant for all four categories, but the magnitude of the influence varies substantially across the categories. In the material to follow we will first describe these differences and then offer interpretations when possible.

Table 6-2: Regression Results for Turnover, Intent to Stay, and Job Satisfaction As Dependent Variables for Full-Time Nurses Under Thirty

	Job Satisfaction				Intent to Stay				Turnover							
Independent Variables	$b^{(1)}$	beta	$b^{(2)}$	beta	$b^{(3)}$	beta	$b^{(4)}$	beta	$b^{(5)}$	beta	$b^{(6)}$	beta	$b^{(7)}$	beta	$b^{(8)}$	beta
Opportunity	.00	.00	-.01	-.01	-.07	-.09	-.05	-.06	.03	.18***	.03	.18***	.03	.15**	.03	.15**
Routinization	-.45	-.33***	-.46	-.34***	.03	.05	.06	.08	-.01	-.04	-.01	-.06	-.01	-.05	-.01	-.05
Participation	.14	.13**	-.15	-.13**	.06	.10*	-.05	-.09	-.01	-.06	-.01	-.05	-.00	-.01	.00	.02
Instrumental Communication	.10	.12**	.10	.12**	.00	.00	-.00	-.00	-.00	-.01	-.00	-.00	-.00	-.00	-.00	-.00
Integration	.05	.06	.05	.07	.03	.08	.01	.04	-.00	-.05	-.00	-.05	-.00	-.02	-.00	-.02
Pay	.00	.01	.00	.03	.00	.02	-.00	-.01	.00	.04	.00	.04	-.00	.04	.00	.04
Distributive Justice	.10	.04	.09	.04	.07	.06	.08	.06	-.01	-.04	-.01	-.04	-.00	-.02	-.00	-.02
Promotional Opportunity	.09	.14**	.08	.12**	.04	.12*	.05	.16***	-.00	-.04	-.00	-.03	.00	.02	.00	.02
Professionalism	-.08	-.03	-.06	-.02	.09	.06	.08	.06	.00	.01	.00	.01	.01	.03	.01	.03
General Training	.45	.10*	.41	.09	-.57	-.25***	-.49	-.21***	-.07	.14**	.07	.14**	.03	.06	.03	.06
Kinship Responsibility	.08	.03	.13	.04	.08	.05	.03	.02	.00	.01	.00	.01	.01	.03	.01	.03
Job Satisfaction					.10	.20***	.11	.21***			-.01	-.07	-.00	-.00	.00	.00
Intent to Stay													-.08	-.34***	-.08	-.34***
Age			-.13	-.08			.05	.06							.00	.02
Length of Service			-.14	-.03			.40	.19***							-.01	-.01
$R^2/\bar{R}^2$	.23	.21	.24	.22	.18	.16	.22	.20	.07	.05	.08	.05	.17	.15	.18	.15

N = 434 (Minimum pairwise N)

N = 467 (Maximum pairwise N)

*p < .05.
**p < .01.
***p < .001.

Table 6-3: Regression Results for Turnover, Intent to Stay, and Job Satisfaction An Dependent Variables for Full-Time Nurses Thirty and Over

Independent Variables	Job Satisfaction				Intent to Stay				Turnover							
	b(1)	beta	b(2)	beta	b(3)	beta	b(4)	beta	b(5)	beta	b(6)	beta	b(7)	beta	b(8)	beta
Opportunity	-.40	-.24***	-.43	-.25***	-.04	-.05	.01	.01	.00	.04	-.00	-.02	-.01	-.05	-.01	-.05
Routinization	-.67	-.43***	-.67	-.43***	.09	.14	.08	.12	.00	.00	-.01	-.11	-.00	-.05	-.00	-.04
Participation	.19	.15*	-.21	-.17**	.03	.07	-.02	-.03	-.01	-.15	-.01	-.11	-.01	-.08	.01	.08
Instrumental Communication	.14	.16*	.15	.17**	-.03	-.07	-.05	-.12	.00	.06	.01	.10	.00	.07	.00	.08
Integration	.03	.03	.04	.04	.05	.14*	.05	.12	.00	.03	.00	.04	.01	.10	.01	.10
Pay[a]	.03	.08	.00	.10	.03	.22***	.00	.17**	-.00	-.11	-.00	-.09	.00	.01	.00	.01
Distributive Justice	-.01	-.01	.01	.00	-.13	-.12	-.15	-.14*	.01	.06	.01	.06	.00	.00	.00	.01
Promotional Opportunity	.11	.15*	.09	.13**	-.01	-.02	.00	.01	-.00	-.03	.00	.01	-.00	-.00	-.00	-.00
Professionalism	-.22	-.07	-.23	-.08	-.10	-.08	-.10	-.08	.01	.08	.01	.06	.00	.02	.01	.03
General Training	.71	.09	.47	.06	-.30	-.10	-.13	-.04	-.00	-.01	.01	.02	-.01	-.03	-.01	-.03
Kinship Responsibility	.91	.20	.89	.19***	.17	.09	.15	.08	-.01	-.05	.00	.00	.01	.04	.01	.04
Job Satisfaction					.16	.39***	.17	.41***			-.02	-.27**	-.01	-.09	-.01	-.09
Intent to Stay													-.07	-.45***	-.06	-.45***
Age			.05	.09			.02	.08							-.00	-.04
Length of Service			-.49	-.13			.37	.23**							.00	.00
$R^2/\bar{R}^2$	.45	.41	.46	.42	.27	.22	.33	.27	.05	-.01	.09	.02	.24	.18	.24	.17

N = 184 (Minimum pairwise N)

N = 203 (Maximum pairwise N)

[a]The unstandardized coefficients for job satisfaction and intent to stay are multiplied by 100.

* $p < .05$.
** $p < .01$.
*** $p < .001$.

Table 6-4: Regression Results for Turnover, Intent to Stay, and Job Satisfaction As Dependent Variables for Part-Time Nurses Under Thirty

	Job Satisfaction				Intent to Stay				Turnover							
Independent Variables	b(1)	beta	b(2)	beta	b(3)	beta	b(4)	beta	b(5)	beta	b(6)	beta	b(7)	beta	b(8)	beta
Opportunity	-.04	-.03	-.07	-.05	-.14	-.18*	-.11	-.14	.05	.31***	.05	.30***	.04	.25***	.04	.22**
Routinization	-.26	-.21**	-.24	-.19***	.03	.04	.03	.04	.01	.09	.01	.04	.01	.05	.01	.05
Participation	.24	.21**	-.27	-.23***	.02	.02	-.01	-.02	.01	.08	.02	.13	.02	.14	-.02	-.13
Instrumental Communication	.12	.16*	.11	.15*	.03	.07	.02	.05	-.03	-.28***	-.02	-.24**	-.02	-.22**	-.02	-.19*
Integration	.04	.05	.06	.08	-.01	-.03	-.02	-.06	.00	.01	.00	.03	.00	.02	.00	.04
Pay[a]	-.03	-.18*	-.00	-.16*	-.01	-.08	-.00	-.09	-.00	-.03	-.00	-.07	-.00	-.09	-.00	-.09
Distributive Justice	-.05	-.02	-.11	-.05	.03	.03	.07	.05	.01	.02	.00	.00	.01	.02	.00	.01
Promotional Opportunity	.10	.15*	.11	.17*	.00	.00	.00	.00	-.01	-.11	-.01	-.08	-.01	-.08	-.01	-.09
Professionalism	.37	.13	.38	.13	-.02	-.01	-.03	-.02	.00	.01	.01	.04	.01	.03	.02	.04
General Training	-.01	-.00	.11	.02	.11	.04	.13	.05	.06	.09	.06	.09	.06	.10	.05	.08
Kinship Responsibility	.23	.06	.22	.06	.66	.33***	.63	.32***	-.05	-.10	-.04	-.09	.00	.01	.01	.01
Job Satisfaction					.13	.24**	.15	.26**			-.03	-.24**	-.02	-.17*	-.02	-.19*
Intent to Stay													-.07	-.29***	-.06	.27***
Age			.28	.18*			-.10	-.11							.01	.03
Length of Service			-.34	-.09			.37	.18*							-.07	-.15
$R^2/\bar{R}^2$	.27	.22	.29	.23	.26	.21	.29	.22	.22	.16	.26	.20	.32	.26	.34	.27
N = 218 (Minimum pairwise N)																
N = 243 (Maximum pairwise N)																

[a]The unstandardized coefficients for job satisfaction and intent to stay are multiplied by 100.

* $p < .05$.
** $p < .01$.
*** $p < .001$.

Table 3-5: Regression Results for Turnover, Intent to Stay, and Job Satisfaction As Dependent Variables for Part-Time Nurses Thirty and Over

	Job Satisfaction				Intent to Stay				Turnover							
Independent Variables	$b^{(1)}$	beta	$b^{(2)}$	beta	$b^{(3)}$	beta	$b^{(4)}$	beta	$b^{(5)}$	beta	$b^{(6)}$	beta	$b^{(7)}$	beta	$b^{(8)}$	beta
Opportunity	-.03	-.02	-.03	-.03	-.06	-.09	-.06	-.08	.01	.05	.01	.05	.00	.01	-.00	-.00
Routinization	-.26	-.21***	-.27	-.22***	-.05	-.07	-.03	-.05	-.00	-.01	-.00	-.04	-.01	-.06	-.01	-.05
Participation	.01	.01	-.01	-.01	-.04	-.07	.04	.07	-.01	-.07	-.01	-.07	-.01	-.10	.01	.09
Instrumental Communication	.30	.41***	.30	.41***	.02	.04	.01	.03	.01	.07	.01	.12	.01	.13	.01	.15
Integration	.01	.02	.02	.02	.01	.03	.00	.01	-.01	-.11	-.01	-.10	-.01	-.09	-.01	-.09
Pay[a]	.02	.12*	.00	.12*	.00	.08	.01	.08	.00	.03	.00	.04	.00	.07	.00	.08
Distributive Justice	-.07	-.03	-.06	-.03	.10	.09	.08	.07	-.02	-.12	-.02	-.12	-.02	-.09	-.12	-.09
Promotional Opportunity	.11	.19**	.10	.19**	-.01	-.02	-.01	-.02	.00	.08	.01	.10	.01	.09	.01	.11
Professionalism	-.42	-.14*	-.43	-.14*	.05	.03	.07	.04	-.01	-.05	-.02	-.07	-.02	-.06	-.02	-.06
General Training	-1.26	-.19**	-1.31	-.20***	-.46	-.13	-.34	-.10	-.02	-.03	-.03	-.05	-.06	-.10	-.06	-.11
Kinship Responsibility	-.21	-.04	-.17	-.04	-.15	-.06	-.23	-.09	-.04	-.09	-.04	-.09	-.05	-.12	-.05	-.12
Job Satisfaction					.14	.27***	.15	.28***			-.01	-.11	-.00	-.01	-.00	-.01
Intent to Stay													-.06	-.36***	-.06	-.36***
Age			.01	.03			-.03	-.12							-.00	-.07
Length of Service			-.13	-.04			.29	.18**							-.02	-.07
$R^2/\bar{R}^2$	.38	.35	.38	.34	.16	.11	.19	.14	.06	.00	.06	.01	.17	.12	.18	.12
N = 161 (Minimum pairwise N)																
N = 171 (Maximum pairwise N)																

[a] The unstandardized coefficients for job satisfaction and intent to stay are multiplied by 100.

* $p < .05$.
** $p < .01$.
*** $p < .001$.

Job Satisfaction As the Dependent Variable

Differences involving seven of the determinants exist when the four categories of nurses are compared for job satisfaction as the dependent variable. Two variables, routinization and instrumental communication, are significant but have different levels of influence for certain categories of nurses. As observed for the total sample, we find for all four categories that the more routinized the work activities, the lower the job satisfaction. (See Column 1 of Tables 6-2 through 6-5.) However, this influence is substantially more important for both age categories of full-time nurses than it is for both age categories of part-time nurses. Increased instrumental communication, for all four categories, operates to increase job satisfaction, but this influence is substantially greater for part-time nurses who are thirty and over.

There are three variables—opportunity, kinship responsibility, and professionalism—which significantly influence job satisfaction for only one category of nurse. In each instance, however, the influence was not expected on the basis of the model. For the full-time thirty-and-over nurses, both greater employment opportunities and higher kinship responsibility operate to increase job satisfaction. Opportunity was expected only to have a direct positive impact on turnover. It is possible, however, for opportunity also to have an indirect positive impact on turnover by decreasing job satisfaction—the results for this one category provide support for this indirect impact. Kinship responsibility was expected to have an indirect positive impact on turnover by increasing intent to stay. Again, it is possible for kinship responsibility also to have a positive indirect impact on turnover by increasing job satisfaction. Finally, professionalism was expected to have an indirect negative impact on turnover through intent to stay. For the part-time thirty-and-over nurses, however, it operates to reduce directly job satisfaction. Once again, it is plausible this variable could also negatively influence turnover indirectly by decreasing job satisfaction.

Findings for general training and pay are contradictory and cannot easily be reconciled with the model. General training, like professionalism, was expected to have an indirect negative impact on turnover through intent to stay. Finding that general training has a negative impact on job satisfaction for the part-time nurses who are thirty and over is not inconsistent with this; like professionalism, general training could have a negative impact on both job satisfaction <u>and</u> intent to stay. For the full-time nurses who are under thirty, <u>however</u>, general training increases, rather than decreases, job satisfaction. This finding is inconsistent with our theoretical expectations. We also expected pay to have an indirect negative impact on turnover through job satisfaction, and this is what is observed for the part-time nurses who are thirty and over. However, pay has a negative impact on job satisfaction for the part-time nurses who are under thirty, another finding inconsistent with the model.

Intent to Stay As the Dependent Variable

One of the most striking differences when the intent-to-stay regression equations (see Column 3) are compared across the four categories is the unique status of the part-time thirty-and-over category. This is the only category of nurse for which job satisfaction is the sole direct cause of intent to stay. In the other three categories, additional variables operate to have direct effects.

There are two instances in which variables have significant effects that were expected, but only for one category. First, only for the full-time under-thirty nurse does general training have a significant net effect (those with baccalaureate degrees have less intention to stay). Second, only for the part-time under-thirty nurse does increased kinship responsibility operate as expected, that is, to increase intent to stay. Finding these effects for only one category each is not surprising, given that these effects were not found for the total sample.

There are five instances where variables not expected to influence intent to stay directly are found to have significant net effects for only one of the four categories. None of these can be viewed as refuting the basic model, however, because the direction of the influence is interpretable within the framework of the model.

Participation, promotional opportunity, integration, and pay were expected to have indirect positive impacts on turnover through job satisfaction, which was, in turn, expected to decrease turnover by increasing intent to stay. However, it is also plausible that these four determinants could indirectly and positively influence turnover by directly increasing intent to stay, and this is what seems to be occurring: increased participation and promotional opportunity operate this way only for the full-time under-thirty nurses, whereas increased integration and pay operate in this manner only for the full-time thirty-and-older nurses. Finally, opportunity was expected to have a direct positive impact on turnover. It is possible, however, for opportunity to influence turnover positively by having a negative impact on intent to stay, as we observe for the part-time under-thirty nurses. In sum, none of these results is actually inconsistent with the model.

Turnover As the Dependent Variable

When turnover is the dependent variable (see Column 7), opportunity operates as hypothesized only for nurses under age thirty. Job satisfaction and instrumental communication are significant only for the part-time nurses who are under thirty. We expected job satisfaction to have an indirect positive impact on turnover through intent to stay rather than through the direct negative impact which we found. Many researchers, however, have hypothesized a direct negative impact of job satisfaction on turnover. We expected instrumental communication to have an indirect negative impact on turnover through job satisfaction and intent to stay; the direct impact on turnover was not expected. The results for job satisfaction, although not specified by the model, are plausible. We cannot, however, understand how instrumental communication could have a direct impact on turnover; it should be mediated by job satisfaction and/or intent to stay, our social psychological variables.

Now that the three dependent variables have been considered, it is instructive to note that distributive justice does not appear as important for any of the four categories of nurses. This is surprising, as this determinant is supported by a fairly substantial body of literature.

Differences in Explained Variance

Not only do we want to know which variables produce variations in turnover, but we also want our model to be able to explain most of the variations in turnover. The results, to this point, have concentrated on differences in the influence of particular variables; we will now focus on explained variance. As before, explained-variance values always refer to the R^2 adjusted for the sample size and the number of variables.

The explained variances for job satisfaction are basically the same <u>within</u> the age categories. The under-thirty nurses, for instance, whether full-time or part-time, have almost identical explained variances, 21 and 22 percent, respectively. However, the explained variances for the thirty-and-over nurses are approximately twice as large, 35 percent for part-time and 41 percent for full-time nurses.

For intent to stay, there is little difference in the explained variances for two categories of nurses, full-time thirty and over (22 percent) and part-time under thirty (21 percent). However, a substantially lower explained variance is obtained for the part-time nurses who are thirty and over (11 percent) and an intermediate value is obtained for the full-time nurses under thirty (16 percent).

Three categories of nurses all have explained variances for turnover which are under 18 percent: full-time under thirty (15 percent), full-time thirty and over (18 percent), and part-time thirty and over (12 percent). The part-time nurses who are under thirty, however, have a substantially larger explained variance (26 percent).

In sum, these data contribute additional support for an argument that the the variables in our turnover model do not operate in the same manner for all categories of nurses.

THE IMPORTANCE OF THE CORRELATES

In Chapter 5 when we discussed the importance of the correlates age and length of service, we identified two ways in which these variables could operate in the model. First, the correlates could be conditioning or specifying variables which interact with the determinants in their influence on turnover. We have, of course, already shown this to be the case, and are, in this chapter, exploring these interactions. Second, the correlates could explain additional variance once the theoretically derived determinants have been allowed to exert their influence. This is still possible even after we have subdivided the nurses by age. Although the variance is reduced for both variables (compare Table 6-1 with Table 5-1), the nurses within each of the four categories still vary on these correlates. This reduction in variation should, however, lead us to expect that the added influence of these two variables, especially age, will be small.

Introduction of age and length of service into the regression equation for job satisfaction (see Column 2) does not significantly increase the explained variance for any of the four categories of nurses, with neither variable having a significant influence. However, for intent to stay as the dependent variable (see Column 4), length of service, but not age, has a significant influence for all four categories of nurses. This is precisely what was observed for the total sample in Chapter 5. When turnover is the dependent variable, neither age nor length of service has a significant net effect for any of the four categories of nurses. Thus, as we observed for the total sample, it is only intent to stay which is better explained by taking into account these correlates.

DISCUSSION

The results of the chapter must now be discussed and interpretations offered. Total causal effects were relied on in discussing the results for the entire sample, and to simplify that discussion, only the larger total effects were considered. However, we will not report and discuss total effects in this chapter because they are based on the standardized coefficients (the betas) and could be misleading, as discussed previously. Instead, we have focused only on the unstandardized coefficients (the b's). To simplify the following discussion, we will focus only on the differences which we are able to interpret meaningfully. The similarities among the nurses will only be briefly summarized because they are consistent with the findings in Chapter 5, where they were discussed.

Similarities

As previously indicated, the following six determinants operated for each of the four categories of nurses as they did for the entire sample: intent to stay, job satisfaction, routinization, participation, instrumental communication, and promotional opportunity. Intent to stay (commitment) reduces turnover, job satisfaction increases intent to stay (commitment), routinization decreases job satisfaction, and participation, instrumental communication, and promotional opportunity produce greater job satisfaction. These similarities provide added confidence in the model with respect to the importance of these six determinants.

Differences

Most of the remaining material in this section will seek to account for the differences we have found among the four categories of nurses. The discussion will deal with each of the dependent variables separately.

Job Satisfaction. Plausible explanations for three differences are possible. The influence of routinization, it may be recalled, was substantially larger for the full-time nurses than for the part-time nurses and, among the full-time nurses, was especially large for the thirty-and-over nurses. These differences are interpretable because of the variations in work-related costs and benefits for the full-time nurses and the part-time nurses. A full-time nurse, for instance, who has a very repetitive job, bears the costs of this work for forty hours per week. However, a part-time nurse, who has an equally repetitive job, only experiences the costs of this work for an average of sixteen hours per week.[5] It is, therefore, no wonder that the negative impact of routinization on job satisfaction is especially pronounced for the full-time nurses.

But routinization is especially important for the full-time thirty-and-over nurses. What could be significant for these nurses is the expected length of time that the costs of repetitive work must be endured. The full-time nurse who is under thirty, who has a very repetitive job, has the possibility of escaping from the job by substituting or adding the variety associated with marriage and having children. Such an alternative is generally not available to the full-time nurse who is thirty and over; this person has a long time to spend in the repetitive work and recognizes the limited potential for altering the routine.

Instrumental communication was observed to be especially important for the part-time thirty-and-over nurses. In addition, and related to our interpretation of this finding, we observed that only for the part-time under-thirty nurses did instrumental communication have a significant influence on turnover. Both of these differences may be interpreted simultaneously. It is comprehensible that instrumental communication would be especially important for the part-time nurses. All nurses need work-related information to perform their job efficiently; the part-time nurses, however, are especially in need of this information because their work patterns remove them from the continual receipt of information, both formal and informal, about the state of their patients. It is not clear, however, why instrumental communication would be especially important for the job satisfaction of the older part-time nurses and the turnover of the younger part-time nurses.

Intent to Stay. Seven differences were found when intent to stay is viewed as the dependent variable, and we can offer reasonable interpretations for four of these differences.

Participation, it may be recalled, was especially important for the older full-time nurses. What seems to be important for these nurses is a difference in values and the distribution of the benefits and costs of work. When all the nurses are asked "how much importance" they attach to making "decisions about" their jobs (Question 11, Appendix A, at the end of the book), the percentages which indicate "Very Important" are as follows: full-time under thirty, 58; full-time thirty and over, 52; part-time under thirty, 60; and part-time thirty and over, 52. The younger nurses thus value participation in work-related decisions more highly than the older nurses. A full-time nurse who is under thirty and who takes an active part in making work-related decisions is receiving a significant benefit, given the higher value placed on this type of activity by the younger nurses. Much less benefit, however, is obtainable for the part-time nurses who are under thirty and who also take an equally active part in making work-related decisions. Participation is, therefore, especially likely to increase intent to stay when it is strongly valued and has sufficient time to make its influence felt. Our model, however, did not predict participation to have an impact on intent to stay; its impact was expected to be on job satisfaction. However, as has been stated previously, it is plausible for participation to influence both job satisfaction and intent to stay—which it does.

The second difference pertains to promotional opportunity, where it was found that this determinant is especially important for the full-time nurses who are under thirty. Long-run costs and benefits associated with promotions seem to be especially critical for this category of nurse. Promotions bring all types of benefits—increased money, greater recognition, and more power—and it is the younger full-time nurses who have more time to experience these benefits than any of the other nurses. Since the older full-time nurses are more established in the hospital and community, promotional opportunities will be less salient in influencing their intent to stay. Since part-time nurses are not likely to be promoted because of their reduced time-commitment to the hospitals, it is not surprising this variable does not affect their intentions to stay. Promotional opportunity is thus likely to increase intent to stay for the nurses who have the best chance of receiving its benefits, the full-time nurses who are under thirty.

Integration was important only for the full-time thirty-and-over nurses. The distribution of costs and benefits again seems to be critical. Close friends at work are the source of many benefits – sociability needs are satisfied, protection is obtained from the organization, information is transmitted, and power is increased. However, it takes time to develop the type of close friendships that maximize those benefits, and it is the full-time nurses thirty and over who have invested the necessary time to develop these close friendships. They have been employed by the hospitals longer than the full-time nurses under thirty (see Table 6-1) and spend more time at work than either of the two categories of part-time nurses. Consequently, it is understandable that the existence of close friends within the organization would be especially likely to increase intent to stay for the older full-time nurses.

The fourth difference pertains to pay, where it was found that this determinant also was important only for the full-time nurses who are thirty and over. This difference is understandable in terms of rising expenses with increased age and the necessity of being adequately reimbursed for time spent at work. Since expenses generally increase with age – mortgage payments must be met, children must be cared for, cars must be purchased, and so forth—the older full-time nurses have more of these expenses than the younger full-time nurses. The full-time nurses, by definition, spend more time at work than the part-time nurses. Since money is a major benefit of working, and since time is a scarce human resource, it is logical that pay is more important for the older full-time nurses than the older part-time nurses. Pay will, in brief, be especially likely to increase intent to stay when expenses are large and investments in work, in terms of time, are substantial.

Turnover. Three differences appeared when turnover was the dependent variable. One of these differences, pertaining to instrumental communication, was discussed when job satisfaction was examined. One of the two remaining differences, that for opportunity, can be given a meaningful interpretation.

It may be recalled that opportunity was important only for the younger nurses. This discrepancy is probably the consequence of differences in general training and discrimination against the older nurses. The younger nurses, for example, are better educated than the older nurses. Means for general training for the four categories of nurses are as follows: full-time under thirty, 1.66; full-time thirty and over, 1.26; part-time under thirty, 1.47; and part-time thirty and over, 1.15 (see Table 6-1). More general education means more long-term potential for taking a variety of jobs and thus more opportunity. In addition, it becomes increasingly difficult to find a job with another employer as one becomes older. The knowledge and skills of older workers become increasingly less transferable to other organizations, and these workers are often excluded from employment consideration (discriminated against) because of this. Opportunity is, therefore, especially likely to increase turnover for younger employees.

Explained Variance. Before attempting to place these similarities and differences in a larger theoretical context, the differences in explained variances must be briefly discussed. About twice as much explained variance in job satisfaction was found for the older nurses. We had hoped Farrell's (1978) research on job satisfaction would be informative here. However, Farrell found just the opposite: considerably more variation in satisfaction was accounted for among those workers with the least amount of work experience. Although age is not perfectly correlated with work experience, and Farrell's measures are not the same as ours, the different results suggest that findings for a broader sample of occupations cannot be used to make generalizations about nurses and vice versa.

The explained variance for intent to stay across the four categories ranges from 11 percent (part-time thirty and over) to about 22 percent (full-time thirty and over and part-time under thirty). We are unable to offer a meaningful substantive interpretation for these differences. As mentioned before, our research was not designed with an awareness of the importance of this variable, and the current literature is not helpful in explaining these differences.

The highest and lowest explained variances for turnover were for the part-time nurses: 26 percent for the part-time under thirty and 12 percent for the part-time over thirty. It is not surprising that the explained variance was the lowest for the older part-time nurses. Most of the research on the determinants of turnover has been conducted on full-time employees, and it could be expected that the model would not adequately explain the turnover of part-time nurses. However, we did not expect the highest explained variance for the younger part-time nurses. Our expectation was that the highest explained variance would be obtained for the full-time nurses. Although it may be shown statistically that this anomalous finding is due largely to the importance of opportunity directly influencing turnover and indirectly influencing it through intent to stay, there is no apparent reason why the model should work best for this category of nurse.

Even though the above differences leave us perplexed, we must emphasize that our examination of the explained variances across the four categories reinforces several of the inferences drawn in the preceding chapter. First, satisfaction is the best-explained variable in all but the category of younger part-time nurses. As in Chapter 5, we interpret this to mean that the more complete literature on job satisfaction (Locke 1976) allowed us to specify the determinants of this variable better than either intent to stay or turnover. Second, as with the total sample, the model does not account for much of the variance in intent to stay for any of the four categories. The need to obtain a better measure of commitment is reemphasized. Third, the introduction of the correlates age and length of service shows again that it is additional determinants of intent to stay which require more investigation. Unknown determinants, indicated by age and length of service, are significantly increasing the explained variance for intent to stay.[6] Finally, the explained variance for turnover is not large for any of the four categories, leading us to the same conclusions and explanations reached in the preceding chapter.

IMPLICATION FOR THEORETICAL APPROACHES

Organizational scholars who study turnover have traditionally not specified their models.[7] Routinization, for example, is hypothesized to influence job satisfaction negatively for all categories of employees. Our results, however, indicated that routinization is substantially more important for the full-time nurses and, among the full-time nurses, was most significant for the older nurses. Although we could not account for many of them, we indicated close to twenty differences among the four categories of nurses similar to the results for routinization. These results support a "contingency approach" to the study of turnover.[8] Future research on turnover must seek to indicate those categories of employees for which the model works the best. In statistical terms, interaction effects must be examined for all determinants of turnover. The contingency approach is widely used in the study of organizations and represents a criticism of the "one best way" approach proposed by classical organizational scholars, such as Frederick J. Taylor. The contingency approach has not been widely used in the study of turnover, and our results supporting this approach constitute some of our most important findings.

We should not, however, overemphasize the extent to which our results support different models of turnover. Similarities do exist among the four categories of nurses. Routinization, participation, instrumental communication, and promotional opportunity generally influence the job satisfaction of the nurses. Job satisfaction increases intent to stay for all categories of nurses. Similarly, increased intent to stay generally reduces turnover. These results support the traditional approach to the study of turnover. Although we found more differences than similarities, thus indicating very strong support for a contingency approach, the results indicate that an either/or choice is not necessary. Just as we previously found that economic <u>and</u> noneconomic determinants are important in the study of turnover, so we now find that there is merit to traditional <u>and</u> contingency approaches to the study of turnover.

This concludes our presentation of results with the individual as the unit of analysis. We first examined the zero-order correlations for the determinants and turnover, then estimated the model for the entire sample, and finally, in this chapter, estimated the model for the four categories of nurses. Our results reported next pertain to the nursing units.

NOTES

1. Some researchers have indicated that there are individual variations concerning the determinants; this topic was discussed in Chapter 2 when we discussed our causal model. Patterned individual variations are an indication that a single model is not appropriate for all populations. However, most of the researchers who study the determinants of turnover have assumed that a single model is appropriate for all populations.

2. The work of Katz (1978) is also relevant at this point. Katz's work stresses the importance of length of service rather than of age.

3. We have no measure of "labor-force experience," which for our study would include length of service plus time spent on other jobs.

4. We use the F test associated with each regression coefficient; significance levels are reported in the tables.

5. Sixteen hours is, of course, two days of work. Some part-time nurses do work more than two days per week; the typical pattern, however, is two days per week.

6. There is, of course, also the possibility that improved measurement of our determinants would increase our ability to explain variance in intent to stay.

7. Footnote 1 is pertinent at this point.

8. A helpful summary and critique of the contingency approach is contained in Schoonhoven (1977). It is more accurate to refer to "contingency approach" than to "contingency theory." No theory is involved in use of this approach, but merely the assumption that conditions must be incorporated into causal models. Additional material about the contingency approach is found in Galbraith (1973), Lawrence and Lorsch (1969), and Woodward (1965).

APPENDIX 6-1

Ideally, to meet the strict statistical requirements of multiple regression, all possible interactions among the independent variables should be tested. In practice, however, this is seldom done, especially when the number of independent variables is more than three or four. There are at least two reasons for this. First, the number of higher-order interaction terms becomes so large that the capacity of most computer programs is surpassed. Second, the intercorrelations among these interaction terms are typically large, thus producing multicollinearity to the extent that interpretation is extremely difficult and matrix inversion is often impossible. For these reasons, as well as the theoretical and practical concerns already mentioned, tests were made only for interactions with amount of time worked, length of service, and age.

Hierarchical testing procedures (Cohen and Cohen, 1975) were used for amount-of-time-worked and age interactions separately from the test of the amount-of-time-worked and length-of-service interactions. The interactions were tested for these variables with only the three theoretically and/or empirically most important independent variables. (For turnover, these were intent to stay, job satisfaction, and opportunity; for job satisfaction, they were routinization, promotional opportunity, and instrumental communication; and for intent to stay, they were job satisfaction, kinship responsibility, and general training.) Even with this reduction in the number of interactions to be checked, difficulty was experienced in testing for the second-order interactions because of multicollinearity among the interaction terms. The standard errors became very large, and some decrements in R^2 were obtained when variables were added to the equations. Thus, it was possible only to test systematically and separately for the first-order interactions of the three variables with age, length of service, and amount of time worked. These first-order interactions were tested net of the additive influence of the other determinants in the model.

When turnover was the dependent variable, both age ($F = 6.20$) and length-of-service ($F = 6.64$) interactions are significant. When intent to stay was the dependent variable, amount-of-time-worked ($F = 4.29$) and age ($F = 3.14$) interactions are significant. When job satisfaction was the dependent variable, amount of time worked ($F = 4.61$) is significant. The degrees of freedom associated with each F ratio are 3 and approximately 1,000.

CHAPTER 7
Analysis of the Nursing Units

This chapter presents the results of estimating the causal model with the immediate work group as the unit of analysis. For this analysis, the scores for the independent variables are obtained by aggregating the scores for all the nurses in a work group, referred to as a "nursing unit," and computing averages. We were able to assign 781 nurses (71 percent of the sample) to 63 nursing units.[1] The score for the turnover variable for each nursing unit is a percentage computed as the number of leavers divided by the number of nurses assigned to the unit and multiplied by one hundred. This measure is similar to what is usually referred to as the "crude turnover rate" (Price 1977, pp. 15-17). The smallest unit contained five nurses; the largest 33. Twelve of the units had between five and nine nurses, while the remaining 51 units had ten or more nurses each.

Prior to presenting the results, it is necessary to discuss how the analysis at the nursing-unit level is different from that at the individual level and how the inferences drawn from one level of analysis cannot automatically be assumed to hold for the other.

DIFFERENT LEVELS OF ANALYSIS: SOME CAUTIONARY NOTES

Initially, it is important to stress the differences in the meaning given the analysis of the nursing units and the analysis just completed, where the individual nurse is the unit of analysis. In this chapter one must think in terms of what it is about the nursing unit that affects the turnover rate for the unit rather than what it is about the nurse that results in a decision to leave or stay in the hospital.

This difference in explanatory orientation may be illustrated by considering any given nursing unit in which some of the nurses are in more routine jobs than others, that is, where there is individual variation on this variable. The results from previous chapters indicate that the nurses in the routine jobs will be least satisfied with their work, and this will result in their intention to leave and a higher probability that they will leave. At the nursing-unit level, however, we can no longer talk about a nurse in a routine job compared with a nurse in a nonroutine job. In fact, for the hypothetical unit discussed above, we are now interested in whether most of the jobs in the unit are routine or nonroutine so that we can compare this unit with the other units where the average "routineness" of the jobs may vary. So the fact that there is a relationship between routinization and satisfaction within the unit is not of relevance. To expand the illustration, we want to know if it is the units which primarily have routine jobs, allow for little participation, are weakly integrated, and so forth which also are the ones with the highest turnover rates. If such data are found, the appropriate way to state such findings would be as follows: a work context (the nursing unit) in which nurses are doing a variety of work activities, are allowed to participate in decision making, are highly integrated, and so forth will produce a higher level of satisfaction and intent to stay among the nurses in the unit and thus will result in a lower turnover rate for that unit.

The differences in interpretation may be further extended to the implications of these findings for policy decisions. Considering only routinization at the individual level of analysis, the objective would be to locate all nurses with routine jobs and attempt to add variety to them. This same relationship at the nursing-unit level, however, would suggest an administrator identify the nursing units with the highest level of routinization and increase the variety in work tasks associated with the jobs in those units.

The statistical literature on why the inferences at one level of analysis cannot necessarily be generalized to other levels has been voluminous (Robinson 1950; Longbein and Lichtman 1978; Firebaugh 1978) and will not be described and discussed here. The major concern in this literature has been whether or not a researcher who conducts the analysis only at the aggregate level can make inferential statements about some less aggregated level of analysis. Since this is not our objective, we will not elaborate on the problems encountered. It is, nevertheless, necessary to speak briefly to some of the problems we will encounter when the results from the individual-unit analysis are compared with those from the analysis to be conducted in this chapter.

Previously, we indicated the problems of comparing standardized coefficients across subpopulations or categories. This is a problem because the standard deviations of the variables differ over these categories. This is also a problem when comparing data analyzed at different levels of aggregation. Therefore, we will have to be cautious about comparing zero-order correlation coefficients and betas for the nursing-unit data with the same coefficients when the individual nurse is the unit of analysis. Whereas the unstandardized coefficients could legitimately be compared across categories (Chapter 6), this may be problematic for analyses conducted at different levels of aggregation. Finally, because the number of "cases" is substantially smaller when the nursing unit is used to analyze the data, use of statistical-significance criteria mean substantially larger coefficients will be required to be significant at the nursing-unit level of analysis. With these cautions in mind, it is instructive to make some comparisons of the descriptive data at both levels of analysis.

Tables 3-5, 3-7, and 7-1 provide means, standard deviations, and zero-order correlation coefficients for the two different units of analysis. The comparison of the means for the variables indicates almost identical values for the individual and nursing-unit data. However, a similar comparison of the standard deviations indicates large differences; in all instances, the standard deviations for the nursing-unit data are smaller than for the individual-level data. This is not surprising, since by using the means for each unit as the data, much of the variation among different nurses within any particular unit is eliminated. As mentioned above, this has implications for the analysis, since standardized coefficients reflect the standard deviations of the variables in the relationship. This effect is easily seen when the correlation coefficients are compared. Column 1, to use as an illustration, displays the zero-order correlations of turnover with all other variables. All of the coefficients, except two, are larger for the nursing-unit data. In fact, in some instances the magnitudes are almost doubled. Generally, the sign remains unchanged except for some instances where the coefficient for the individual-level data is essentially zero. These patterns hold for most of the other correlations in the table. Although these differences in correlations serve to illustrate that aggregated and unaggregated data often produce different correlations for the same variables, this point can be made even more dramatically by comparing the same correlation when the data are aggregated at the hospital level. At the individual level, the correlation between job satisfaction and turnover is -.12, but when the hospital is the unit of analysis (the data are aggregated for each hospital), it is .69. More is said about the hospital data in Appendix 7-2 at the end of this chapter.

The points we have attempted to make in this section may be summarized as follows: (1) the substantive interpretation of the results from the two levels of analysis is not the same, and (2) comparisons of the results at the two levels must be made with caution.

THE ZERO-ORDER CORRELATIONS

Considering only the correlations of job satisfaction with all other variables (Table 7-1) except for intent to stay and turnover, we find ten of the 14 coefficients meet the significance criterion, and of these the directions of six match expectations.[2] Assuming the same causal ordering as for the individual level of analysis, the six correlations indicate that the level of satisfaction in nursing units is increased by reducing the repetitiveness of the work activities, increasing the participation in job-related decision making, increasing the job-related information transmitted to the nurses, more closely linking the effort expended on the job with the money received, providing the opportunity to advance in the job hierarchy, and including more older nurses in the unit.

Unexpected were the correlation indicating that the nursing units with the most-satisfied nurses are also the units where the pay is low, the nurses have fewer close friends, and the nurses are less professional in orientation. The nursing units with the most-satisfied nurses are also the units where there is a higher concentration of part-time nurses. Since there is little research relating job satisfaction and amount of time worked, we had no expectations regarding this relationship.

Seven of the 15 correlations with intent to stay meet the significance criterion, and all but one of these are consistent with our expectations. The average intent to stay of the nurses in a unit is increased by the amount of job-related information transmitted to the nurses, reducing the number of nurses with general training, including nurses who have greater kinship responsibilities, and increasing the level of job satisfaction of the nurses in the unit. The average intent to stay of the nurses is also increased when the nurses are older and have been employed in the hospital for a longer period of time. As with job satisfaction, we had not expected the units composed of nurses with the lowest intent to stay to have a higher concentration of full-time nurses.

The examination of the correlations of turnover with all other variables indicates that eight of the 16 coefficients are greater than .21. The direction of five of these is consistent with our expectations. The nursing units with the highest turnover rates are characterized by a high concentration of nurses who have the greatest job opportunities outside the hospital, little communication of work-related information, high concentrations of generally trained nurses, nurses with weak intentions to stay and a

Table 7-1: Correlation Matrix for All Variables: Nursing-Unit Data[a]

	1	2	3	4	5	6	7	8	9	10	11	12	13	14	15	16	17
1	--																
2	-.179	--															
3	-.472	.240	--														
4	.330	-.165	-.008	--													
5	.006	-.007	-.474	-.087	--												
6	-.128	.096	.465	.085	-.178	--											
7	-.223	.296	.468	-.093	-.236	.349	--										
8	.225	-.190	-.261	-.045	-.108	.076	-.068	--									
9	.282	-.144	-.224	.246	-.105	-.019	-.012	.264	--								
10	-.154	.120	.274	-.155	.196	.032	.083	-.314	-.281	--							
11	-.137	.043	.405	-.142	-.110	.332	.405	.018	-.219	.266	--						
12	.205	.045	-.224	.167	-.199	-.157	-.148	.271	.163	-.305	-.111	--					
13	.318	-.293	.196	.234	.076	.255	.032	.089	.009	-.032	.257	-.132	--				
14	-.167	.434	.125	-.130	-.117	-.150	.206	-.233	-.386	.162	.005	.198	-.281	--			
15	.219	-.262	-.299	.129	.021	-.026	-.064	.346	.750	-.353	-.034	.132	.071	-.536	--		
16	-.141	.484	.225	-.113	-.007	-.184	.161	-.319	-.221	.275	.030	.091	-.314	.456	-.407	--	
17	-.153	.454	-.044	-.229	.002	.226	.220	-.191	-.223	.068	-.120	.161	-.641	.549	-.413	.586	--
Mean	.202	6.37	28.29	11.24	12.08	13.78	26.42	8.79	$8,802	6.99	21.40	1.92	1.30	4.91	.61	29.11	3.13
St. Dev.	.121	.75	1.81	1.07	1.68	1.56	2.00	1.92	$1,494	.65	2.95	.71	.26	.53	.19	4.84	.50

[a]Correlations $\geq \pm.21$ are statistically significant at $p < .05$; correlations $\geq \pm.25$ are statistically significant at $p < .01$.

NOTE: 1 = Turnover; 2 = Intent to Stay; 3 = Job Satisfaction; 4 = Opportunity; 5 = Routinization; 6 = Participation; 7 = Instrumental Communication, 8 = Integration, 9 = Pay, 10 = Distributive Justice; 11 = Promotional Opportunity, 12 = Professionalism, 13 = Education, 14 = Kinship Responsibility, 15 = Amount of Time Worked, 16 = Age, 17 = Length of Service.

strong dedication to high professional standards.

We did not expect, however, that the units with the highest turnover rates would be composed of nurses with the highest pay and with more close friends in the hospital. Finally, we did not have expectations about the turnover rates of units with different compositions of full-time nurses and part-time nurses, so we did not expect that having more full-time nurses in the unit would be associated with high turnover rates; if anything, the reverse might have been expected.

It also is instructive at this time to examine the relationship of the two correlates age and length of service with the other variables, as was done in Chapter 5. With regard to age, we have already discussed that the nursing units where the average job satisfaction and intent to stay is highest will also be the units with the oldest nurses. We learn from the other correlations that the units with the oldest nurses are characterized by higher levels of distributive justice, a lower concentration of generally trained nurses, and nurses who have more kinship responsibilities. We also observe that these same units are characterized by lower average pay and lower integration.

For length of service, we find, as expected, that the nursing units which are composed of nurses with the greatest work experience are characterized by greater distributive justice, more instrumental communication, fewer generally trained nurses, less opportunity outside the hospital, and more kinship responsibilities. We did not expect, however, that these same units also would be characterized by low pay and low participation.

As with the data previously reported (Chapters 4-6) using the nurse as the unit of analysis, we must be careful not to overinterpret these zero-order data. Multivariate analysis must be conducted where variables are controlled and net effects can be examined.

RESULTS: REGRESSION AND PATH ANALYSIS

The results from the regression analysis are contained in Table 7-2. Although we eventually will want to contrast our findings at the individual level (Chapter 5 and 6) with these nursing-unit data, our attention initially will be focused only on the standardized regression coefficients.

The first regression equation (see Column 1 of Table 7-2), the regression of job satisfaction on all determinants except turnover and intent to stay, results in six statistically significant determinants: routinization, participation, integration, instrumental communication, distributive justice, and general training. These findings for routinization, participation, instrumental communication, and distributive justice are consistent with the model. We would expect the level of job satisfaction in a nursing unit to decrease as the work in the unit becomes increasingly repetitive. Similarly, we would expect the level of satisfaction to be greatest in the units whose nurses are the most involved in job-related decision making, who provide the most information relevant to doing the job correctly, and who reward the nurses fairly for the effort expended.

The findings for the influence of integration and general training are not consistent with the model, however. Integration was expected to decrease the turnover rate indirectly by exerting a positive impact on level of job satisfaction; we find instead a negative impact–nursing units composed of nurses who have more close friends are also the units where the level of job satisfaction is the lowest. General training was expected to increase turnover indirectly through a negative impact on intent to stay–and such an impact was found. If general training is also to have an indirect impact on turnover through job satisfaction, and such an impact is plausible, then this impact would be expected to be negative. It is posi-

Table 7-2: Regression Results for Turnover, Intent to Stay, and Job Satisfaction As Dependent Variables

Independent Variables	Job Satisfaction				Intent to Stay				Turnover							
	$b^{(1)}$	beta	$b^{(2)}$	beta	$b^{(3)}$	beta	$b^{(4)}$	beta	$b^{(5)}$	beta	$b^{(6)}$	beta	$b^{(7)}$	beta	$b^{(8)}$	beta
Opportunity	-.04	-.02	-.04	-.02	-.06	-.09	-.06	-.08	.02	.20	.02	.20	.02	.16	.02	.18
Routinization	-.51	-.47***	-.51	-.47***	.14	.30+	.10	.23	-.00	-.01	-.00	-.03	.01	.09	.00	.01
Participation	.27	.24*	.30	.26*	.05	.10	.08	.17	-.01	-.17	-.01	-.16	-.01	-.12	-.00	-.04
Instrumental Communication	.17	.19+	.17	.19+	.05	.14	.04	.10	-.01	-.12	-.01	-.12	-.00	-.06	-.01	-.18
Integration	-.20	-.21*	-.16	-.17+	-.01	-.03	-.00	-.00	.01	.16	.01	.15	.01	.14	.01	.16
Pay[a]	-.01	-.07	-.01	-.10	.01	.15	.00	.08	.00	.20	.00	.20	.00	.26	.00	.18
Distributive Justice	.52	.19+	.41	.15	-.10	-.09	-.10	-.09	.01	.04	.01	.05	.00	.01	.01	.06
Promotional Opportunity	.05	.08	.04	.06	-.01	-.03	-.01	-.05	-.00	-.05	-.00	-.05	-.00	-.06	-.00	-.08
Professionalism	-.19	-.07	-.25	-.10	.11	.10	.04	.04	.02	.10	.02	.10	.02	.14	.01	.07
General Training	1.14	.16+	1.07	.15	-.81	-.29*	-.48	-.17	.16	.34*	.16	.35*	.11	.24+	.22	.48**
Kinship Responsibility	-.11	-.03	-.17	-.05	.45	.31+	.38	.26	.00	.02	.00	.02	.03	.14	.02	.09
Amount of Time Worked	-.94	-.10	-.52	-.05	-.42	-.10	.10	.03	-.03	-.04	-.03	-.04	-.06	-.09	.09	.14
Job Satisfaction					.14	.34+	.10	.24			-.00	-.03	.01	.10	.01	.10
Intent to Stay													-.06	-.40**	-.07	-.46**
Age			.09	.24*			.04	.27+							.00	.08
Length of Service			-.39	-.11			.11	.07							.11	.45*
$R^2/\bar{R}^2$	.65	.57	.68	.59	.37	.20	.42	.23	.33	.16	.33	.15	.42	.26	.50	.32
Nursing Unit Data (N=63)																

[a]The unstandardized coefficients have been multiplied by 100.

+ $p < .10$.
* $p < .05$.
** $p < .01$.
*** $p < .001$.

tive, however, indicating that a nursing unit's level of job satisfaction is increased by changing the composition of the unit to include more nurses with general training.

When intent to stay is regressed on all determinants except turnover (see Column 3), four determinants are statistically significant: job satisfaction, kinship responsibility, routinization, and general training. Only the results for routinization are inconsistent with the model.

We expected increased job satisfaction and greater kinship responsibility to produce greater intent to stay: nursing units composed primarily of nurses who like their jobs and who have the most local kinship responsibilities also have the nurses with the highest average intent to stay (increased commitment, we would like to say). We also expected increased general training to produce reduced intent to stay: nursing units with strong concentrations of generally trained nurses also have nurses who least intend to stay.

The model indicates that routinization is expected to have an indirect negative impact on turnover through job satisfaction. It is plausible for routinization also to have a negative impact through intent to stay; the literature only explicitly suggests the impact through job satisfaction. If routinization is to influence turnover through intent to stay, however, its impact should be negative rather than positive, as we find in this analysis: in the nursing units where the work is highly repetitive, the nurses express the strongest intent to stay. This finding becomes even more puzzling because routinization has the expected impact on job satisfaction. There is also little difference in the magnitudes of the four coefficients. Based on the model, we would expect the coefficient for routinization to be considerably lower than the coefficients for the other three determinants. Routinization again confounds our expectations.

Two determinants–intent to stay and general training–are statistically significant when turnover is regressed on all variables in the causal model (see Column 7). The results for intent to stay are consistent with the causal model: nursing units composed of members who mostly intend to stay have, as a result, lower turnover rates. Since we view intent to stay as a dimension of commitment, this means that nursing units with highly committed nurses have low turnover rates. General training was expected to increase turnover indirectly through intent to stay. These regression data indicate that general training increases turnover, but its impact is direct: nursing units with high percentages of baccalaureate nurses have higher turnover rates. This direct impact of general training on turnover is a puzzle; its impact should have been indirect through one of our social psychological variables, intent to stay or job satisfaction. This and other puzzles will be examined in the discussion section which follows this presentation of the results.

Finally, of the two significant variables, intent to stay is a more important determinant of turnover than general training. The beta coefficient for intent to stay is slightly more than one and a half times the size of the coefficient for general training. The greater importance of intent to stay is expected, since its impact on turnover is believed to be direct.

The Role of Correlates

When age and length of service are entered into the regression equations, a significant increase in explained variance is not obtained for either job satisfaction or intent to stay, but is obtained for turnover. The increases for job satisfaction, intent to stay, and turnover are, respectively, .03, .05, and .08 (see Columns 2, 4, and 8 of Table 7-2). For the turnover equation, it is only length of service which has a significant effect, however. The positive coefficient indicates that net of other variables, the turnover rates are highest in the nursing units with a higher concentration of more experienced nurses. As discussed in previous chapters, we interpret this to mean that other analytic constructs related to length of service must be sought in attempting to explain turnover.[4]

Explained Variance

The explained variances of interest, as before, are the adjusted R^2s. They are, for job satisfaction, intent to stay, and turnover, respectively, .57, .20, and .26. What is most striking about these data is the high value for job satisfaction relative to the other two. As at the individual level of analysis, our model better explains job satisfaction than intent to stay and turnover.

Path Analysis

Figure 7-1 presents the path diagram representing the results contained in Table 7-2. The coefficients in the figure and table are slightly different because the path diagram is based on equations using only the statistically significant variables. A discussion of the diagram is not necessary since it reflects, in an abbreviated form, the data in Table 7-2, which we have already reported.

The Role of the Intervening Variables

As with our analysis at the individual level, the importance of job satisfaction and intent to stay as intervening variables is observed for the nursing-unit data. This is evident in several different ways.

First, an examination of the path diagram in Figure 7-1 shows that almost all of the variables do not directly affect turnover but instead operate through job satisfaction, intent to stay, or both.

Second, by examining the changes in R^2 values (unadjusted) in Table 7-2, we observe that intent to stay, overall, is a more important variable than job satisfaction in explaining variation in turnover. Comparing Column 5 and Column 6 shows that adding job satisfaction to the equation does not increase the explanatory power. However, by then adding intent to stay (compare Columns 6 and 7), we observe an increase of about .10.

Third, making the same regression-equation comparisons, but looking at the beta coefficients instead, we can determine the degree to which the coefficients for the causally prior variables are reduced by including the intervening variables. Making this comparison for Columns 5 and 6, we observe very little change, indicating that job satisfaction is not serving a very important mediating role. Comparing Column 6 with 7 does show somewhat larger changes for several variables, indicating that their influence is in part indirect through intent to stay. (Note especially the coefficient for general training, which is reduced from .34 to .23, indicating that about 36 percent of its causal influence is through intent to stay.)

Total Effects

The total effects on turnover for all the determinants are contained in Table 7-3. Arranged by order of magnitude, the determinants are as

Figure 7-1: Path Model for Nursing-Unit Data

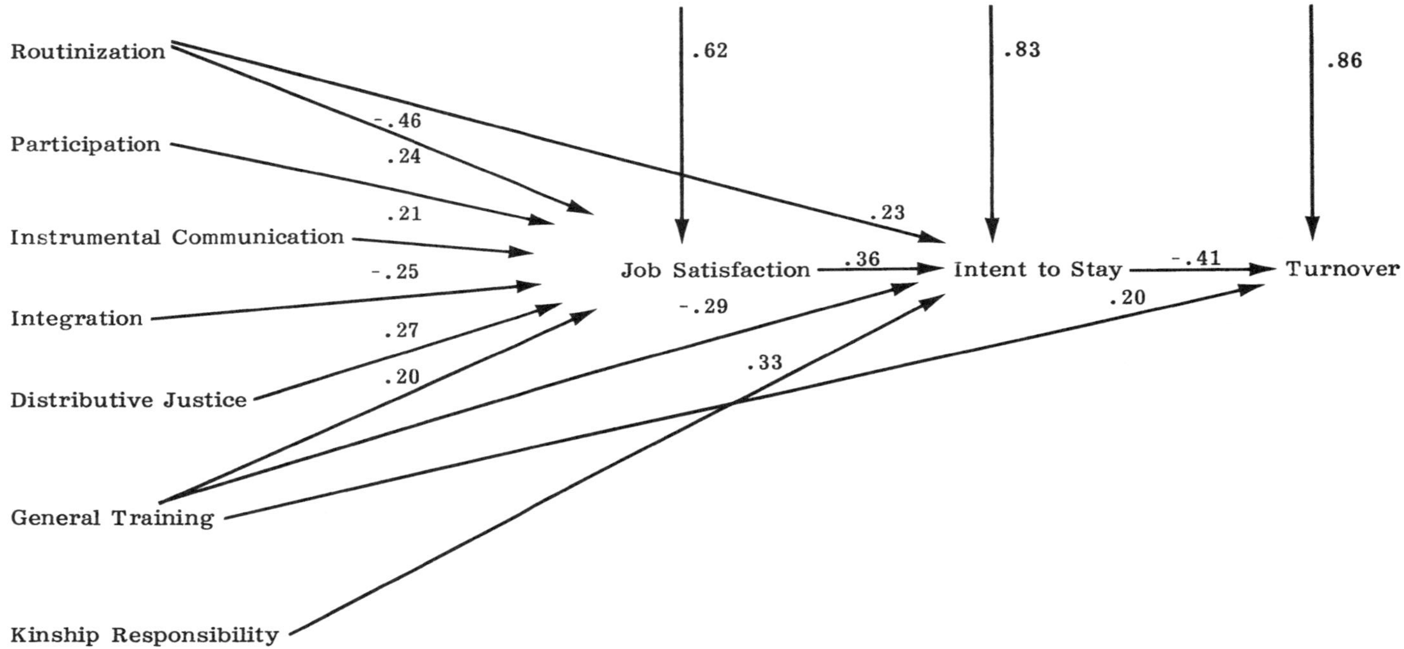

follows: intent to stay (-.41), general training (.29), job satisfaction (-.15), kinship responsibility (-.14), distributive justice (-.04), participation (-.04), integration (.04), instrumental communication (-.03), and routinization (-.02). The direction of some of the indirect linkages are inconsistent with what we had expected; they will be examined in the discussion section.

Table 7-3: Direct, Indirect, and Total Effects for Nursing Units

Variables	Direct Effects	Indirect Effects Via: Job Satisfaction	Indirect Effects Via: Intent to Stay	Indirect Effects Via: Job Satisfaction and Intent to Stay	Total Effects
Intent to Stay	-.41	--	--	--	-.41
Job Satisfaction	ns[a]	--	-.15	--	-.15
Opportunity	ns	ns	ns	ns	ns
Routinization	ns	ns	-.09	.07	-.02
Participation	ns	ns	ns	-.04	-.04
Instrumental Communication	ns	ns	ns	-.03	-.03
Integration	ns	ns	ns	.04	.04
Pay	ns	ns	ns	ns	ns
Distributive Justice	ns	ns	ns	-.04	-.04
Promotional Opportunity	ns	ns	ns	ns	ns
Professionalism	ns	ns	ns	ns	ns
General Training	.20	ns	.12	-.03	.29
Kinship Responsibility	ns	ns	-.14	ns	-.14

[a]Not statistically significant.

DISCUSSION

Most of what we have observed at the nursing-unit level of analysis is consistent with our model as presented in Chapter 2. The turnover rate of a nursing unit will be reduced if the intent to stay of the nurses in the unit can be increased. This level of commitment will be increased directly if the nurses in the unit can be made more satisfied with their jobs and if fewer baccalaureate nurses are hired for the unit. The level of job satisfaction will be increased if the work activities are made less routine, the nurses are allowed to participate more in decision making, are provided with more work-relevant information, and are paid fairly in terms of the amount of energy expended on the job.

As described in an earlier section, four findings are inconsistent with our expectations. First, the direct positive path from routinization to intent to stay was not expected. It suggests that units which allow less variety in work activities generate a greater intent to stay among the nurses. What is perplexing about this finding is that routinization does operate as expected by exerting a negative influence on job satisfaction. We initially reasoned that this might be due to the different full-time/part-time compositions of the nursing units. However, given that this variable is controlled (see Columns 3 and 4), this explanation is inappropriate. The data in Column 4 do indicate that when age and length of service are controlled, the influence of routinization, although still positive, is no longer statistically significant. We are unable, however, to offer a meaningful substantive interpretation of this.

Second, although integration was expected to influence job satisfaction only directly, as we find, we expected its influence to be positive. The negative coefficient indicates that if the nurses in a unit are allowed to form more friendships with other nurses in the hospital, the level of satisfaction of the nurses in the unit will decrease. The only plausible explanation we could arrive at has to do with how integration was measured; it refers to the number of close friends in the hospital rather than in the nursing unit. (See Appendix A at the end of the book.) If we had measured this for the nursing unit, then the expected positive effect might have been found.

The final two inconsistencies exist for the general training variable. As Table 7-2 and Figure 7-1 indicate, this variable has a significant net effect on all three of the dependent variables. As we expected, nursing units with a higher concentration of nurses with more general training also have nurses with the highest average level of intent to leave the hospital. However, we also found that units with a higher concentration of nurses with a general training are also the units in which the nurses exhibit the highest level of job satisfaction. Nurses with a general training (that is, baccalaureate nurses) are taught the professionally preferred nursing procedures by colleges and universities; when they begin work in hospitals, it is likely that their new working environment will not measure up in many important ways to the nursing procedures stressed by colleges and universities–the result should be reduced job satisfaction.[5] We do not have a ready explanation for the relationship we did observe.

Finally, although we expected turnover to be higher in the units with the greater concentration of generally trained nurses, we did not expect the influence to be direct, as we observe. We expected general training to increase turnover through a negative impact on intent to stay. Had we conceptualized intent to stay as commitment, and had we available the promising and newly developed index of commitment developed by Porter and his colleagues (Mowday et al. 1979), the coefficient for commitment might have been considerably higher and, when controlled, might have reduced the coefficient for general training. It is unlikely that all of the determinants will operate only indirectly on turnover through a barely adequate measure of commitment. Support for this line of reasoning is obtained when Column 6 is compared with Column 7. The beta coefficient for general training is reduced from .35 to .24 when intent to stay is included. It is plausible that the Porter measure of commitment will reduce general training's direct impact on turnover to statistical insignificance. Only future research can check this reasoning.

COMPARISON OF THE RESULTS AT THE TWO LEVELS OF ANALYSIS

The literature on turnover has not clearly distinguished between theory and analysis strategies for different levels of analysis. Scholars in turnover research have not taken care to ask whether or not their models are appropriate for both individual and aggregate levels of analysis. The research we have reported here is unique because we have the opportunity to determine empirically whether a model, developed primarily to account for why particular individuals leave and others stay, adequately identifies the determinants of the turnover rate of nursing units in a hospital.

Previously in this chapter we warned the reader about drawing inferences about one level of analysis from the results of another, and even about making comparisons of results across different levels of aggregation. Because of this, we will not directly compare magnitudes of corresponding coefficients at the two levels, but will instead discuss general similarities and differences.

The major difference between the two sets of results is the larger amount of explained variance (for all three dependent variables) at the nursing-unit level of analysis. Based on this, it would be tempting to argue that the model we have proposed is a "better" representation of reality at the nursing-unit level. We will cautiously allow for this interpretation, but will also remind the reader that research on aggregated data rather consistently results in larger correlations among variables and hence larger explained variances. (The data we report at the hospital level in Appendix 7-2 lend support to this general finding.) Other differences are that (1) opportunity and chances for promotional advancement are only important at the individual level, whereas integration is important only at the aggregate level, and (2) some of the direct and indirect linkages among the variables are not the same at the different levels of analysis.

Overall, the results from the two levels of analysis are quite similar: (1) the major net determinant of turnover is intent to stay; (2) the major net determinant of intent to stay is job satisfaction; (3) the major net determinant of job satisfaction is routinization; (4) the model explains best the variance in job satisfaction, followed by intent to stay and turnover; (5) the signs of the coefficients of corresponding pairs of variables in the final model are the same; and (6) job satisfaction and intent to stay are shown to be important intervening variables.

The results lead us to conclude that our turnover model is appropriate for both levels of analysis and that the results at one level would not greatly mislead anyone interested in the other level. Additional data are presented in Appendices 7-2 and 7-3. Appendix 7-2 presents correlational data on how the variables in the model are related when the hospital is the unit of analysis. Appendix 7-3 presents a contextual analysis which provides information on whether contextual characteristics of the nursing units, hospitals, and communities have an influence on the likelihood the nurse will leave the hospital. In general, these additional analyses do not lead us to alter the conclusions just stated.

NOTES

1. The remaining 29 percent of the nurses are excluded from the analysis.

2. The statistical-significance criteria are presented in footnotes to the tables. In the regression analysis, we used a .10 level of significance.

3. See Appendix 7-1 of this chapter for an analysis of the importance of several other variables not included in the original causal model.

4. Also, as previously indicated, our measurement of constructs must be improved.

5. Many nurses do not, of course, accept these "professionally preferred nursing procedures." It is, however, the colleges and universities

which generally determine, in the long run, what are professionally acceptable procedures in nursing.

6. Most of the literature about the impact of size on turnover uses the organization as its unit of analysis. This would be the hospital in our research. Sometimes, however, the immediate work unit is used to analyze the data (Muchinsky and Tuttle 1979). We thus decided to use size of the nursing unit to estimate the causal model at this point. The nursing unit is the immediate work group for the nurses in our study.

We know of no literature which indicates that inequality per se is a determinant of turnover. Our reason for using inequality as a possible determinant is described in the following paragraph in the text.

Shift pattern as a possible determinant was suggested to us by Price's pilot study (Price and Bluedorn 1979). Most of the nurses seemed to prefer working the same shift rather than rotating among the day, evening, and night shifts. We are aware of no literature which suggests that shift pattern might be a determinant of turnover.

7. The reference here is to the relationship between size of the organization and turnover (Price 1977, pp. 89-90). Muchinsky and Tuttle review some studies which indicate (1979, p. 63) that size of work unit may be positively related to turnover.

8. The nursing units, for example, vary greatly by the extent of routinization. Scores for the units can, of course, be averaged to obtain a routinization score for a hospital. Such scores, however, should be viewed with caution, due to the large variation among the nursing units. What is true for routinization also applies to the other determinants of turnover.

9. Our inclusion of religious affiliation and size of community is based on our sociological background. Sociologists view these characteristics as important determinants of behavior.

APPENDIX 7-1

As discussed by Longbein and Lichtman (1978), it is not unusual to find that in analysis at the aggregate level, variables are important which are not important at a lower level of aggregation. Although it is desirable to identify such variables through the development of theory, it also is possible to engage in some exploratory research to identify them. Such is the case for what we report here. We attempted to determine the importance of three variables in explaining the turnover rate: the size of the unit, the extent of salary inequality in the unit, and the shift pattern (straight or rotating) used in the unit.[6] The measure for each of these and the results are presented below.

The magnitude of salary inequality was measured by a Gini index (Allison 1978). This is a standard measure used in stratification and economics to assess the level of inequality among cases comprising some particular social unit; the higher the score, the greater the magnitude of inequality. It may be viewed as an objective measure of inequality, whereas our measure of distributive justice purposefully gauges the individual nurse's assessment of the extent to which his/her work activities are fairly rewarded. It may be remembered that at both the individual and the aggregate levels of analysis, distributive justice was not an important determinant of turnover. The inequality variable does not necessarily tap the same phenomenon as distributive justice, however. Just because there exists extreme inequality does not mean the nurses view the unequal distribution as unfair. Similarly, a small degree of inequality may be viewed as unfair if nurses believe their relative inputs are different. Drawing from the general principles of stratification theory, we would expect that the turnover rate would be the highest in a unit where there is the greatest salary inequality. In general, we argue that people do not approve of extreme inequality (Lipset 1963) and will attempt to avoid settings in which it exists.

The zero-order correlation coefficients of the Gini index with several variables of interest are as follows: distributive justice (.22), job satisfaction (.15), intent to stay (.07), and turnover (-.11). Only the correlation with distributive justice is statistically significant, and it tells us that in nursing units where the salary inequality is the greatest, the nurses perceive the distribution of rewards to be the fairest. Thus, as suggested above, little inequality in rewards does not necessarily mean the individuals approve of it. The coefficients with job satisfaction, intent to stay, and turnover are not statistically significant, so no attempt will be made to interpret the signs of these coefficients. Given these low correlations, the findings for the regression analysis are not surprising. Adding the inequality variable to the equations represented by Columns 2, 4, and 8 in Table 7-2 produces very small and statistically nonsignificant regression coefficients. In short, the magnitude of salary inequality in a nursing unit does not operate to influence directly or indirectly the level of job satisfaction, the level of intent to stay, or the turnover rate.

The shift composition of a unit was measured as the proportion of nurses in the unit who were working straight shifts as opposed to those working rotating shifts. Nurses who work "straight" shifts always work the same hours; they do not regularly work ("rotate") on the day, evening, and night shifts. Our expectation was that the turnover rates would be highest where the rotating shifts predominated. The correlations of this shift variable with the three dependent variables are as follows: job satisfaction (-.12), intent to stay (-.12), and turnover (-.04). None of these correlations is statistically significant.

Adding the shift variables to the equations represented by Columns 2, 4, and 8 in Table 7-2 produces statistically significant coefficients for job satisfaction and intent to stay, but not turnover. The beta when job satisfaction is the dependent variable is -.20 ($p < .05$), indicating that net of the other variables, nursing units with the highest percentage of nurses working straight shifts exhibit the lowest levels of job satisfaction. The beta when intent to stay is the dependent variable is -.27 ($p < .05$). This tells us that nursing units with the greatest number of straight shifts also have nurses with the lowest levels of intent to stay. Since job satisfaction influences the turnover rate indirectly and intent to stay directly, we may conclude that the shift composition of a nursing unit operates indirectly to affect the turnover rate. In particular, having a higher concentration of rotating shifts decreases the turnover rate. We have no explanation for this finding.

Finally, we measured size by the number of nurses in the unit. Given the ambiguous nature of the literature concerning the relationship between size and turnover, we had no expectations about the turnover of the different-sized units.[7] Several relevant zero-order correlations are as follows: job satisfaction (.07), intent to stay (.17), and turnover (-.17). None of these is statistically significant, however, Adding size of unit to the equations represented by Columns 2, 4, and 8 in Table 7-2 results in small and statistically nonsignificant regression coefficients.

In sum, although we were able to identify three variables which had not been included in our original model, and for which plausible arguments could be made for their importance at the nursing-unit level, two of these variables do not operate to influence the turnover rates of nursing units either directly or indirectly. The shift composition does operate indirectly through job satisfaction and intent to stay, however.

APPENDIX 7-2

The Hospital As the Unit of Analysis

When we emphasized early in this chapter the problems associated with making inferences about individuals on the basis of aggregated data, we reported some correlation coefficients computed on data aggregated at the hospital level to illustrate our argument. We do not want to leave the impression that there is something inherently wrong with analysis at the aggregated level; it can provide useful and informative data, as long as inference limitations are understood.

With this in mind, we now offer a brief discussion of the correlations among the variables in the model after we have aggregated the individual-level data to obtain means on all variables for each hospital. These means then serve as the variable scores for each of the seven hospitals. Because there are only seven cases, a correlation coefficient must be very large for it to be statistically significant. In addition, the small number of hospitals will not allow us to use multiple regression to estimate partial coefficients of the turnover model because there are more variables than cases. We will, nevertheless, be able to make some statements about how various characteristics of hospitals are related to the turnover rates of these hospitals. Table 7-4 displays the zero-order correlations which are statistically significant at the $p < .10$ level.

The correlations of variables with level of job satisfaction provide mixed support for expectations. Consistent with expectations is the positive correlation of age; it indicates that hospitals with the highest level of job satisfaction among the nurses are characterized by a higher concentration of older nurses. Inconsistent with expectations is the correlation of general training with job satisfaction. We find that the hospitals with the most satisfied nurses are the ones where there is a higher concentration of baccalaureate nurses. In addition, we find the hospitals with the most satisfied nurses also are the hospitals where the nurses participate more. Finally, we observe that it is the hospitals with the highest concentration of part-time nurses and where the job opportunities are the greatest that also have the nurses who are most satisfied with their jobs.

We find the hospitals with the nurses having the highest level of intent to stay are also the ones with lower concentrations of nurses with long length of service records. The finding is inconsistent with what we had expected.

Examination of the variables significantly related to turnover also indicates mixed findings with respect to our expectations. As expected, we find it is the hospitals where the level of intent to stay is low and where there are more baccalaureate nurses that have the highest rates of turnover. However, and inconsistent with our expectations, we find that the turnover rate is highest in the hospitals characterized by a high level of job satisfaction and a higher concentration of older nurses.

We offer no interpretation of these data for the following reasons. First, seven hospitals is not a large enough sample to allow for conclusions we would be willing to stand behind. Second, data about the relationships among these variables at the hospital level must be questioned on at least two grounds; one concerns how the variables were measured. In many instances, the organizational characteristics measured are more applicable to nursing units than to hospitals.[8] We can question, then, whether aggregation of these data results in measures of hospital characteristics. The second concerns the policy implications which can be drawn from this research. We expect it would be more practical to attempt change at the nursing-unit level than at the hospital level. More is said about this in the final chapter.

Table 7-4: Statistically Significant Correlations Among Variables Aggregated at the Hospital Level

Variables	Correlation	Significance Level
Turnover-Intent to Stay	-.82	<.05
Turnover-Job Satisfaction	.68	<.10
Turnover-General Training	.75	<.05
Turnover-Age	.79	<.05
Intent-Length of Service	-.82	<.05
Job Satisfaction-Opportunity	.69	<.10
Job Satisfaction-Participation	.79	<.05
Job Satisfaction-General Training	.92	<.01
Job Satisfaction-Age	.79	<.05
Job Satisfaction-Full/Part Time	-.90	<.01
Opportunity-Instrumental Communication	-.82	<.05
Opportunity-General Training	.80	<.05
Routinization-Pay	.86	<.05
Routinization-Distributive Justice	.69	<.05
Participation-Age	.67	<.10
Participation-Full/Part Time	-.76	<.05
Instrumental Communication-Promotional Opportunity	.74	<.10
Instrumental Communication-Kinship Responsibility	.77	<.05
Integration-Age	-.80	<.05
Promotional Opportunity-Kinship Responsibility	.67	<.10
General Training-Age	.72	<.10
General Training-Full/Part Time	-.75	<.10
Age-Length of Service	.69	<.10
Age-Full/Part Time	-.76	<.05

N=7

APPENDIX 7-3

Contextual Analysis

We wish to expand on some of the issues raised in this chapter and to consider the suggestion that an explanation of individual variation in turnover requires the inclusion of both individual and social-system-level variables. There has been among social scientists a longtime concern with what are typically called "contextual effects" (Blau 1960b; Lazarsfeld 1959; Riley 1964). It is argued that to account adequately for an individual's behavior, the researcher must not only examine characteristics of individuals but also investigate the influence of the various social contexts of which the individual is an integral part. For example, there has been recent interest (Alwin 1974; Alexander and Eckland 1977) in whether the educational context (measured by such variables as the school's social-class composition, racial composition, student/teacher ratio, and so forth) has an influence on the student's cognitive development, aspirations for more education, occupational achievement, and so forth. Although much of this research has been critically and negatively assessed (Hauser 1972), there still remain interest and appropriate methods for assessing the existence of such contextual effects.

Hauser shows (1972) that it is possible to determine the magnitude of contextual effects without directly measuring and including them in the regression model. The procedure involves using dummy (binary) variables to represent the social units, which, in turn, represent the contexts expected to produce the effects. The variance contributed by this set of dummy variables is an upper limit on the influence any such contextual effects can have.

Applying the strategy directly to our turnover data, we wish to determine whether the likelihood a nurse will leave a hospital is influenced by the contextual characteristics of (1) the nursing unit, (2) the particular hospital, (3) the affiliation (Protestant or Catholic) of the hospital, and (4) the community in which the hospital is located.[9]

Table 7-5 shows that the maximum effect that nursing-unit contextual variables can have is a statistically significant 11 percent (uncorrected) of the total explained variance in turnover. However, the real "test" of whether unit contextual effects should be investigated further must be based on the variance-explained net of the individual-level determinants examined in Chapters 4-6 (Hauser 1972). Table 7-5 shows a net R^2 value of about 7 percent, which is not statistically significant, however. This indicates that specific unit contextual variables (e.g., unit size and salary inequality) need not be examined in attempting to account for turnover.

We also determined whether the nursing-unit context influences the nurse's job satisfaction and intent to stay. It is found to account for about 18 percent of the variance in job satisfaction and 13 percent in intent to stay, both being statistically significant. Although this contribution is reduced when the determinants are controlled, the contribution of the unit contextual effects is still statistically significant, thus indicating that there may be something about the particular unit in which the nurse works that contributes (above and beyond the variables in our model) to job satisfaction and intent to stay.

We also considered the possibility that the work environments in Protestant- and Catholic-affiliated hospitals are diverse enough to result in differences in turnover, job satisfaction, and intent to stay. Without controls for other variables, this context effect is statistically significant only for turnover. In addition, it remains significant when the determinants are controlled. This finding tells us that the turnover rates for Catholic- and Protestant-affiliated hospitals are different. We learn that nurses are more likely to leave Catholic-affiliated hospitals than Protestant-affiliated hospitals, even after all other determinants are controlled.

In addition to exploring the effect of the religious affiliation of the hospital, we examined the possibility that each hospital provides a unique

Table 7-5: R^2 Values for Regression Equations Used in the Contextual Analysis

	Context Variables			
	Hospitals	Prot.-Cath.	Community	Units[a]
Job Satisfaction As Dependent Variable				
Independent Variables				
(1) Determinants[b]	.2790*	.2790*	.2790*	.3181*
(2) Context[c]	.0174*	.0030	.0043	.1755*
(3) 1 + 2	.2963*	.2794*	.2810*	.4118*
(4) 3 - 1	.0173*	.0004	.0002	.0937*
Intent to Stay As Dependent Variable				
Independent Variables				
(1) Determinants[b]	.2531*	.2531*	.2531*	.2707*
(2) Context[c]	.0056	.0005	.0014	.1287*
(3) 1 + 2	.2612*	.2533*	.2553*	.3560*
(4) 3 - 1	.0081	.0002	.0022	.0853*
Turnover As Dependent Variable				
Independent Variables				
(1) Determinants[b]	.1890*	.1890*	.1890*	.1853*
(2) Context[c]	.0170*	.0059*	.0024	.1076*
(3) 1 + 2	.2010*	.1941*	.1901*	.2573*
(4) 3 - 1	.0120*	.0051*	.0011	.0720

[a] Results are based on the 781 nurses in units composed of more than five nurses.

[b] The determinants are: opportunity, routinization, participation, instrumental communication, integration, pay, distributive justice, promotional opportunity, professionalism, general training, kinship responsibility, amount of time worked, job satisfaction, intent to stay, age, and length of service.

[c] As described in the text, there are 6 dummy variables representing the 7 hospitals; one dummy variable representing the Protestant-Catholic distinction; two dummy variables representing the three communities; 63 dummy variables representing the 64 nursing units.

*The R^2 or the increment in R^2 is significant at $p < .05$.

work environment which has an independent influence on the three dependent variables in the model. The data in Table 7-5 indicate that this possibility exists only for job satisfaction and turnover; about 2 percent of the variance in each is accounted for by hospital differences. Even after controls for other variables, these hospital effects remain statistically significant. To reiterate, this means that after we control for the determinants in the model, we are better able to account for individual variation in both turnover and job satisfaction by taking into account the particular hospital in which the nurse works.

Finally, we considered the possibility that the community environment has an independent influence on the three dependent variables. With regard to turnover, finding such an effect could be interpreted to reflect different job-opportunity structures across the three communities included in the study. The data show, however, that community effects do not exist, with or without controls for the other variables.

To summarize, these findings suggest the possibility of contextual effects associated with the nursing units (on job satisfaction and intent to stay), with religious affiliation of the hospital (on turnover), and with the hospitals (on job satisfaction and turnover).

We will now attempt to give some substantive interpretation of these findings. We believe that results for the influence of hospitals and the religious affiliation of hospitals do not merit such an effort, however. The additional explained variance by religious affiliation is a mere .5 percent, and for hospitals it is under 2 percent. Thus, we argue that attempts to identify and measure specific contextual effects associated with religious affiliation or the hospitals per se would be a waste of energy. Such specific contextual variables, whatever they might be, will not aid us substantially in explaining any of the three dependent variables.

However, given that we can explain an additional 9 percent of the variance in job satisfaction and intent to stay by allowing for unit contextual effects, we conclude that further investigation of these possible effects is warranted. In an attempt to determine what it is about the nursing units which influences a nurse's job satisfaction and intent to stay, we introduced two new variables which measure nursing-unit characteristics. The first was size, which measures the number of nurses in the unit, and the second is a Gini index (Allison 1978), which is a measure of the salary inequality in a unit. These variables were added separately and together to the regression models, which already include the determinants in the model. In no instance, however, did either of these variables contribute significantly in explaining variance in turnover, job satisfaction, or intent to stay at the individual level of analysis.

These results of contextual analysis lead us to conclude that either other unit contextual variables must be identified and measured or, as we discussed in previous chapters, more attention must be given to improving the research design and measures at the individual level of analysis. We believe the latter strategy will be the most fruitful.

CHAPTER 8
Summary and Recommendations

This final chapter will summarize the major findings, suggest specific steps to reduce the turnover of hospital nurses, indicate improvements for future research which seeks to explain variations in turnover, and conclude with some final thoughts about the research.

THE MAJOR FINDINGS

The findings will be presented separately for the two units of analysis, the individual and the immediate work groups. Since the similarities outweigh the differences, and because it is easier to make general recommendations based on similarities among the nurses, we will not summarize the differences which we found among the four categories of nurses.

The Entire Sample

Five determinants were especially important when the individual was used as the unit of analysis: intent to stay, opportunity, general training, job satisfaction, and kinship responsibility.[1] The determinants whose increase resulted in reductions in turnover were intent to stay (which we view as a dimension of commitment), job satisfaction, and the existence of local kin. The determinants whose increase produced greater amounts of turnover were many available jobs outside the hospitals and training which prepared the nurses to operate in diverse occupational settings.

The Four Categories of Nurses

Six determinants were important for at least three categories of nurses: intent to stay, job satisfaction, routinization, participation, instrumental communication, and promotional opportunity. The determinants whose increase produced less turnover were as follows: intent to stay, job satisfaction, participation in making job-related decisions, the receipt of work-related information, and the chance to get ahead occupationally in the hospitals. Increased repetitiveness of work resulted indirectly in greater turnover.

The Nursing Units

Four determinants were significant when the immediate work group was used as the unit of analysis: intent to stay, job satisfaction, kinship responsibility, and general training.[2] When nursing units are composed of nurses with high average levels of intent to stay, job satisfaction, and the existence of local kin, then these units are, as a consequence, likely to have low rates of turnover. Nursing units with high percentages of baccalaureate nurses, however, are likely to have, as a result, high rates of turnover.

RECOMMENDATIONS TO REDUCE TURNOVER

When making recommendations designed to reduce the turnover of nurses employed by hospitals, we are tempted to establish priorities based on the magnitudes of the total effects of the determinants, as given in Tables 5-3 and 7-3. Following this strategy, we would conclude that intent to stay is the most important determinant, which would lead us to recommend that hospital administrators attempt to increase the level of this variable before any other variables are altered. Continuing with this strategy, our second recommendation would be to increase the level of job satisfaction; the third would be to decrease job opportunities, and so forth. Utilizing the magnitudes of total effects or regression coefficients to rank order variables for purposes of policy recommendations is not an appropriate strategy, however. First, there are statistical reasons for not using this kind of information for such a purpose.[3] Second, practical recommendations, that is, recommendations which can be implemented without great cost, are not possible for a number of the variables in our model.

To elaborate on this second point, let us consider intent to stay and job satisfaction, both of which are intervening variables in the causal model. Simply telling hospital administrators to increase levels of these will be neither very helpful nor very practical. It is necessary to identify explicitly the measures which must be taken to alter these variables. Our model and data, in fact, indicate how this could be accomplished: the six determinants which directly influence job satisfaction and/or intent to stay should be altered. For example, reducing routinization, increasing participation, reducing general training, and so forth will have this effect, since these variables have indirect effects on turnover through job satisfaction and intent to stay. In the pages to follow we will describe in detail how these particular changes might be implemented. Opportunity is another variable which was found to be quite important but which, for practical reasons, will not be included in our discussion of recommendations. Although reducing job opportunities for nurses will result in reduced turnover, it is unrealistic to assume hospital administrators have the power to influence the number of nursing jobs available in the environment.

Before we discuss our recommendations, a cautionary note is necessary. The recommendations we make should not be expected to result in drastic reductions in turnover. There are two reasons for this. First, as already discussed, our model explains 17 percent of the variance in turnover, meaning that manipulation of the variables in the model will not result in even a moderate level of control over turnover. Second, by not being able to make practical recommendations about the direct manipulation of job satisfaction and intent to stay, we reduce the possibility of controlling the nursing turnover. This is true because (1) neither of the variables is completely explained by the causally prior determinants (which we recommend should be manipulated), and (2) intent to stay has a substantial effect of its own (the direct causal path) even after we take into account the indirect effect of the six determinants and job satisfaction through it. In practical terms, this means that it would be advisable to increase both job satisfaction and intent to stay in ways other than by manipulating the six determinants we found to be important. Our data do not, however, allow us to identify how this might be done.

Five additional preliminary comments are pertinent regarding the recommendations. (1) Seven of our eight recommendations are based on the findings of our research; the final recommendation is based on the measurement research of Van der Merwe and Miller (1976). (2) Suggestions about how to implement the recommendations will be mostly ignored. Our recommendations will differ greatly in the ease of their implementation: some can be implemented easily, whereas others–for legal, financial, or administrative reasons–can be implemented only with considerable difficulty, if at all. Legal considerations are very important; the law must be scrupulously obeyed in implementing the recommendations. (3) A cost-benefit perspective is essential when considering the recommendations. All of the recommendations involve both costs and benefits. We assume that the benefits will be substantially greater than the costs, especially over a period of several years. (4) It should be emphasized that quality patient care, not the reduction of turnover, is the goal of the hospitals we studied. Turnover, as was emphasized in the introductory chapter, does result, in some instances, in improvement in patient care. We assume, however, that excessive turnover is harmful to the patients and costly for the hospital. And it is excessive turnover that we believe should be reduced. (5) Finally, the recommendations are not arranged by order of importance. The first recommendation, for instance, will not result in greater reduction in turnover than the eighth recommendation. Since the recommendations are based on the six determinants, we arbitrarily use the sequence of the determinants in the tables to order the recommendations.

Eight recommendations, or sets of recommendations in most instances, will be advanced. (1) Allow voluntary transfers between nursing units. (This recommendation is based on the findings concerning routinization.) Nurses with specialized training are often assigned to units, because of the staffing needs of the hospital when they are hired, where they have little or no opportunity to make use of their special skills and knowledge. Still other nurses develop special interests, extended and deepened by extra education of various types, which are underutilized by the hospitals. Transfer among nursing units would permit better use of these specialized skills and knowledge. Both the nurses and the patients should benefit by such transfers. Some of the complaints about repetitive work seem to be the result of insufficient use of specialized skills and knowledge.

Such transfers must, of course, be voluntary. If the nurses are not willing to transfer, then such movement constitutes a punishment and will decrease job satisfaction and commitment. One has only to note the hostility to "pulling" among nurses–involuntary transfers for one shift–to appreciate the necessity of keeping the transfer voluntary.

A policy of allowing transfers requires that vacancies throughout the nursing department be officially posted in some manner. Many nurses will learn about forthcoming vacancies informally. Such channels, however, are not too reliable and are often unfair. Information transmitted informally is not always accurate, and the information is often kept among a few close friends. Organization, therefore, should depend primarily upon formal means to transmit information about vacancies.

The mechanics of such transfers should not be too difficult to manage. A nurse in a specialized unit (such as cardiac intensive care) resigns, the vacancy is officially posted throughout the nursing department, the resigning nurse is replaced by a nurse already employed (in a general medical unit, for instance), and finally, a new nurse is hired to fill the vacancy created by the nurse who is transferred.

To allow voluntary transfers among nursing units is not to institute a system of "musical chairs" among the nurses. Too-frequent transfers would be just as harmful as allowing no transfers.

(2) Hold regular and brief meetings of the nursing units during working hours. (The findings concerning participation and instrumental communication are the basis of this recommendation.) "Regular" means scheduled at a specific time. The frequency of the meetings will naturally vary for the different units, but once each week seems to be sufficiently regular. The scheduling of the meetings should be arranged so that the maximum number of part-time nurses can attend because these are the individuals for whom the meetings will be especially important. Brief meetings are essential because of the needs of the patients and the cost of staff time. Seldom should the meeting last longer than about forty-five minutes.

"Unit meetings" refers to assembling all, or substantially all, of the members of a unit at a specific place. Individual meetings, between the unit supervisor and a staff nurse, for instance, are important but are not an adequate substitute for unit meetings. Since there are three shifts of nurses, there will have to be three meetings of each unit. This will require two extra visits to the hospital by the unit supervisor, but it is more fitting to inconvenience the supervisor than the staff nurses since the conduct of meetings is a responsibility of the supervisor.

These meetings constitute a pressure to communicate work-related information and to allow participation in making work-related decisions. A unit supervisor, for example, who meets regularly with the members of the unit will be constrained by the pressure of the group to share information and to allow greater participation in operation of the unit. The meetings also provide an opportunity for supervisors to receive information from the staff nurses and for the staff nurses to communicate with one another. Upward and horizontal communication is as important as downward communication.

All organizations must, of course, plan for the regular transmission of work-related information. Such transmission, however, is particularly difficult to bring about adequately in hospitals because of the constant pressure to care for sick patients, the regular arrival and departure of patients, the necessity of three different work shifts, and the mixture of full-time workers and part-time workers. Hospitals thus must make a special effort to do what is much easier for other organizations.

The mere existence of unit meetings, of course, does not guarantee better communication or greater participation in decision making. A minimum of information may be communicated and the meetings may allow for no sharing of power. The quality of the meetings is all-important: without a genuine sharing of information and power, the meetings may be too costly to be a regular feature of hospital operations. Unit supervisors must know how to conduct meetings so that information and power are shared.

(3) Promote primarily from within the nursing department. (Our findings regarding promotional opportunity are the basis for this recommendation.) This type of promotional policy allows maximum use of existing opportunities for promotion. The present career structure allows for relatively few promotinal opportunities for nurses; these limited openings should be reserved primarily for the currently employed staff. Implementation of such a policy will naturally require an official posting of vacancies

for the existing staff before outsiders are notified.

Hospitals cannot, of course, promote entirely from within. Situations sometimes arise when the existing staff does not possess the needed qualification or when an outsider possesses clearly superior competence. These situations are, however, relatively rare. When higher positions, mostly "nursing-unit supervisor," are available within the nursing department, the burden of proof should be on the person who wishes to hire an outsider.

(4) Create an alternate career structure for staff nurses. (This recommendation is based on our findings regarding participation and promotional opportunity.) A career is a succession of related and ranked occupations through which persons move in a predictable sequence.[4] The occupations in a career are ranked in terms of money, prestige, power, rights, and responsibilities. The only career available to most hospital nurses consists of the following sequence of occupations: staff nurse, unit supervisor, assistant nursing director, and nursing director. Most notable is the fact that this career consists mostly of administrative positions; only the lowest position, that of staff nurse, is primarily professional.

There might, for instance, be four steps in an alternate career for staff nurses: staff $nurse_1$ through staff $nurse_4$. Each step should result in a significant increase in money, prestige, rights, and responsibilities. Without these increases, a genuine alternate career does not exist. Administrative rights and responsibilities will probably increase somewhat as a nurse progresses through the sequence of occupations. What is essential, however, is that each occupation in the sequence consist of primarily professional rights and responsibilities. What we are proposing is a "professional career structure" for hospital nurses.

Pay and number of people supervised will not always be correlated if an alternate career structure is implemented. Some of the experienced staff $nurse_4$'s, for example, will make more money than an inexperienced nursing director. Or again, many, perhaps most, of the staff $nurse_4$'s will make more money than the unit supervisors. An alternate career structure thus departs in some instances from a "civil-service type of organizational structure" in which pay is always correlated with the number of people supervised.

Advanced training, such as possession of a master's degree, should not be a prerequisite for movement to the position of staff $nurse_4$; nor should possession of any specific type of education be preferred, such as having a baccalaureate degree. What is absolutely basic is ability; there should be a steady progression of ability as a nurse as one moves from staff $nurse_1$ to staff $nurse_4$. For a hospital to have a genuine alternate career structure, there should also be sizable distributions of nurses throughout the sequence. One or two staff $nurse_4$'s in a large hospital, for instance, hardly constitutes a genuine alternate career structure.

An alternate career for staff nurses would create more opportunity for promotion within the hospital. Although this system would be espeically attractive to the full-time nurses who are under thirty, the system would also be attractive to the other three categories of nurses. An alternate career would mean that a staff nurse need not become an administrator to receive significant increases in money, prestige, power, rights, and responsibilities; such benefits would be enjoyed by remaining a staff nurse. Implementation of this recommendation would also seem to be especially important in view of the greater proportion of women who work full-time for longer periods of their life. The recommendation is thus consistent with what seems to be major change in the role of women in American society. Since an alternate career structure would mean more power for the top of the career structure, the staff $nurse_3$ and the staff $nurse_4$, the result should be less dissatisfaction about making job-related decisions. The nurses who are strongly motivated to participate in making job-related decisions will probably be staff $nurse_3$'s and staff $nurse_4$'s. These nurses are now relatively powerless staff nurses.

(5) Recruit more diploma nurses. (The results about general training are the basis for this recommendation.) This recommendation must be qualified by the fact that most of the nurses in the sample (71 percent) were diploma nurses. Only 16 percent of the nurses had baccalaureate and/or graduate degrees; the remaining 13 percent of the nurses were trained as associates.

Nurses with baccalaureate and/or graduate degrees would naturally continue to be hired. Their links with universities provide a source of new ideas and an emphasis on professionalism that hospitals can ill afford to lose. The recommendation means simply that if turnover is to be reduced, relatively more of the nursing staff should be diploma nurses.

The first recommendation is contrary to the current emphasis on baccalaureate training as the preferred course for nurses. Reduced turnover is, of course, not the goal of hospitals. It may be that patient care is, in the long run, improved by greater emphasis on baccalaureate training. We believe this to be the case. We also believe that adjustments are required by both the hospitals and the baccalaureate nurses if the quality of patient care is to be improved. Our study, however, focuses only on turnover, and the results indicate that nurses with baccalaureate training have higher rates of turnover than nurses without such training. One cost of the current emphasis on baccalaureate training will probably be more turnover. This cost, to emphasize a point previously made, must be weighed against the many long-term benefits for the patients which are likely to result from an increased emphasis on baccalaureate training.

(6) Hire more local nurses who are married and who have children. (Our findings about kinship responsibility are the basis for this recommendation.) A local nurse is one who has been born and reared in the community in which the hospital is located. Local nurses are likely to have parents and siblings living in the area, and these relatives constitute a constraint not to leave the hospital. Marriage and children also create additional relatives, which further constrain turnover. In addition to the kinship responsibility created by all of these relatives, these nurses are also likely to have close friends working in the hospital. These close friends will generally be the result of long residence in the community and will constrain turnover slightly.[5]

Aggressive recruiting will be necessary to locate local nurses who are married and who have children. Many of these nurses will have left the labor force and will not respond to the typical newspaper advertisement. The existing staff of nurses within the hospital will generally be aware of these nurses in the community and can serve as valuable aids in recruiting.

Since many of these nurses will have left the labor force, they will commonly require special training before they can start working again. Local public schools, such as community colleges, should provide regular refresher courses for nurses, since the benefits of such training will accrue to no single work organization. Hospitals cannot be expected to provide costly training that will benefit other organizations that might employ the nurses who have taken the refresher courses. Even with refresher courses provided by community colleges, these nurses will require extra training by hospitals. The hospitals may also have to provide extra flexibility in working hours to accomodate these nurses. There is nothing sacred about three eight-hour shifts. This extra training and flexible scheduling will be costly for the hospitals. Our view is that these costs will be less than the considerable benefits received by the lower turnover of these nurses.

Competence must not, of course, be compromised by this recommendation. When competence levels are approximately equal, preference should be given to local nurses who are married and who have children.

None of the recommendations in this section, it should be emphasized, are intended to suggest violation of merit criteria in the recruitment, promotion, and retention of nurses. Weakening of merit criteria threatens the provision of quality care for patients, and such weakening is unacceptable.

(7) Hire more nurses who are over thirty. (Age is not, of course, part of our causal model. Correlates, however, can be used as the basis of recommendations.) The rate of turnover decreases sharply for the older nurses: part-time under thirty, 30 percent turnover; full-time under thirty, 24 percent; part-time over thirty, 11 percent; and full-time over thirty, 8 percent. The rate of turnover for all the nurses is 20 percent.

Previous comments about the local nurses who are married and who have children are also applicable to the nurses thirty and over. Aggressive recruitment will be needed to locate and hire these nurses; and once hired, extra training will be necessary, since many of them will have been out of the labor force for some time. The extra costs, however, should be less than the benefits because of the reduced turnover among these nurses.

Nurses under thirty will naturally continue to be hired. The recommendation means that if other things are approximately equal, especially competence, then preference should be given to the older nurses.

(8) Obtain better data about turnover. Most hospitals calculate crude turnover rates for their nursing departments. The number of leavers during a period, usually a year, is divided by the average number of nurses employed during the period. A common way of obtaining the average number employed is to add the number employed at the beginning and end of the period and divide by two. Crude turnover rates are also calculated for nursing units within the nursing department.[6]

The crude turnover rate is a helpful measure because it indicates the volume of turnover experienced. And the greater the volume, the greater the cost. Hospitals, however, should also calculate the median length of service for all nurses who leave.[7] The median is better than the arithmetic mean because the distribution of leavers is highly skewed. Most of the leavers, for instance, consist of short-service nurses. With the median length of service for the leavers, the hospital will know where nursing turnover is occurring, in terms of length of service. It makes a big difference, for example, whether or not turnover is occurring among the long-service nurses or the short-service nurses. Costs are greater and the quality of patient care is more threatened by the turnover of long-service nurses. The median length of service of the leavers is thus an excellent complement to the commonly used crude turnover rate.

Care should be exercised in calculating these rates for small nursing units. The turnover of a single nurse will make a major difference in either of these statistics with small units. If the size of the unit is less than twenty, this fact should be noted and the rates should be viewed with caution (Van der Merwe and Miller 1976, p. 57).

To summarize, we suggest eight steps that hospitals can take to reduce the turnover of their nurses: the hospitals can allow voluntary transfers among nursing units; hold regular and brief meetings of the nursing units during working hours; promote primarily from within the nursing department; create an alternate career structure for staff nurses; recruit more diploma nurses; hire more local nurses who are married and who have children; hire more nurses who are over thirty; and obtain better data about turnover by calculating the median length of service for all nurses who leave as a supplement to the commonly used crude turnover rate.

Three final comments are in order before making recommendations for future research. First, it is likely that a single individual will possess several qualities emphasized by these recommendations. A local nurse who is married and who has children is also likely to be a diploma trained nurse who is thirty or over. Such a nurse thus satisfies three of the recommendations. Each recommendation, however, should separately contribute toward the reduction of turnover. Second, no recommendations were made about full-time nurses and part-time nurses because these two categories of nurses had almost identical rates of turnover (full-time nurses, 20 percent turnover, and part-time nurses, 19 percent). These facts are important because there is little knowledge about these two categories of nurses in the turnover literature. One might think that rates of turnover would be considerably higher among the part-time nurses, but such is not the case in our research. Only further research will determine the extent to which our findings can be generalized. Third, the recommendations and the results must be viewed separately. The recommendations, if implemented, should reduce turnover. It is possible, however, that some of the recommendations will have unanticipated costs which will nullify the intended benefits. In addition, the manner of implementing the recommendations is all-important. Sound recommendations based on the very best data can have basically harmful effects on the hospital if they are clumsily implemented. Finally, other recommendations can be devised which may even more adequately implement the policies indicated by the empirical data. It is essential that the recommendations we have made not be viewed as the only ones which could be derived from our empirical findings.

FURTHER RESEARCH

Recommendations to improve further research on the determinants of turnover will be discussed under two headings, theory and data-methods.

Theory

At least three improvements are needed in our causal model. (1) It might be worthwhile to distinguish two categories of leavers, those who leave the labor force and those who seek work elsewhere. Different parts of the model may work differently for these two categories of leavers. Pay, for instance, may not deter a nurse who leaves the labor force to rear a family; pay, however, may have prevented the turnover of a career nurse who leaves for more money and better fringe benefits at another hospital. This is, of course, consistent with the contingency point of view that we have adopted toward the study of the determinants of turnover. Such a distinction will require intensive study of larger hospitals in major metropolitan areas. Only an intensive study can provide the needed data, and only large hospitals in major metropolitan areas will have enough turnover to make such a distinction meaningful.

(2) Intent to stay should be replaced by commitment, conceptualized as loyalty toward the organization. Porter and his colleagues view (Mowday et al. 1979, pp. 225-226) commitment as consisting of three components: a strong belief in and acceptance of the organization's goals and values; a willingness to exert considerable effort on behalf of the organization; and a strong desire to maintain membership in the organization. Our intent to stay corresponds to their third component. We suggest that each of these components is part of what is usually meant by loyalty toward the organization. Loyalty is a more abstract way to refer to the three components and is thus a more parsimonious way to conceptualize commitment.

(3) Three additional determinants should be added to the model.[8] The model includes all major determinants commonly cited in the literature

except size (Price 1977, pp. 89-90).[9] Our hospitals are all basically of medium size, so we could not determine the influence of size. We started our research without grant support, and we chose easily accessible hospitals to maximize our sample of nurses, with the result that all of our hospitals were basically the same size.

Another determinant which has some support in the literature is effectiveness, the extent to which organizational goals are achieved.[10] Although sparse, the literature seems to support consistently the idea that increased effectiveness reduces turnover.[11] Effective organizations are successful in obtaining scarce resources which can be used to reward their members, and often create a sense of pride in work well done, which is a form of job satisfaction.

We would also like to suggest a third determinant, for which we can find no support in the literature but which has occurred to us a result of our two studies of nursing turnover. This determinant is kinship priority and is the relative importance assigned to the kinship system. A nurse who resigns her job to accompany her husband to a new community assigns higher priority to the kinship role of wife than to the occupational role of nurse. Or an executive who declines a promotion because it would require his wife to leave a good job (the "dual-career family") is, in this instance, assigning higher priority to the kinship role of husband than to the occupational role of executive. We believe that strong kinship priority reduces turnover for both males and females.[12]

Kinship priority is, in our view, a different concept than kinship responsibility. The latter concept refers to the existence of local kin, whereas the former concept refers to the importance assigned to the kinship system. Kinship responsibility is thus an environmental variable, whereas kinship priority is a social psychological variable. Although kinship priority is an individual evaluation, it typically is socially prescribed. Females in American society, for instance, have been socially expected to assign greater importance to kinship roles than to occupational concerns.[13]

Our expectations are mixed regarding the explanatory power that may be added by these three additional determinants. The literature citing size as a determinant is unclear and it is not likely to be an important determinant. Price used effectiveness in his pilot study (Price and Bluedorn 1979), and it was not an important determinant, so it was not used in our research.

We are more hopeful regarding kinship priority. Intensive interviews with nurses who have quit hospitals, plus our knowledge of sex roles in American society, strongly suggest the importance of kinship priority as a determinant. Many married nurses leave hospital employment because they assign greater priority, as is prescribed by American society, to kinship roles than to occupational roles. A married nurse who works in a hospital and whose husband takes a job in another community is socially expected to resign her job to accompany her husband to the new community. And most nurses conform to social expectations, that is, they resign their positions in the hospital.

The problem is that we have had difficulty measuring kinship priority. Price constructed a crude measure in his pilot study, and it did not turn out to be an important determinant. We also, unsuccessfully, sought to devise a measure of kinship priority for this study.[14] If an adequate measurement can be devised, we believe that kinship priority will be an important determinant of turnover.

Data and Methods

We can think of at least seven procedural improvements needed in future research on the determinants of turnover. Since these needs have mostly been discussed when the results were presented, the material can be briefly summarized.

(1) The most important need is to shorten the period of time between data collection for the independent and dependent variables. We believe that our explained variance was considerably reduced because we had to wait fourteen months to collect the turnover data from the time we measured our independent variables. Six months would be a more preferred interval.

(2) The organizations studied should be located in a large metropolitan area. It is only in such areas that one is likely to obtain sufficient turnover to reduce to six months the period of time between measurement of the independent and dependent variables. Turnover seems to be considerably higher for organizations located in large metropolitan areas (Moffatt and Hill 1970; Russell 1968).

(3) Organizations of different size should be studied. This procedural modification is, of course, needed if size is to be included in the causal model, as the previous section suggested. With organizations of different size it should also be possible to obtain considerable variations in size of work units The estimated model should include size of both organizational and work units.[15]

(4) Males and females should be included in future research. We suspect that some of our findings may be the result of the fact that all of our nurses were females. Pay, for instance, may have been somewhat reduced in importance because most of our nurses probably were not primary wage-earners. In addition, kinship responsibility may have been as important as it was because kinship obligations have traditionally been of higher priority to females than to males. The only way to check for these possibilities is to include both males and females in the same sample.

(5) The occupations selected to be studied should exhibit greater variance with respect to professionalism. The nurses studied, it may be recalled, were almost all at the low end of the professional continuum. If professionalism operates as a determinant, this would not have been evident in the results, due to the lack of variance on this variable. Greater variation, for example, could have been obtained by studying all the nursing personnel–assistants, licensed practical nurses, and registered nurses.

(6) The independent variables should be measured at more than one point in time, We only measured the independent variable once, in August, 1976; the data collected at this time were then used to explain variations in turnover in October 1977. We could order our independent and dependent variables chronologically, since the former were measured before the latter. Although job satisfaction and intent to stay were ordered as intervening variables, we relied on theory and statistical procedure to justify this. Two measurements are probably the most that can be reasonably made on our independent variables, since respondents resist completing the same questionnaire too many times. Measures at two points in time, however, would provide greater assistance in chronologically ordering our independent variables.

(7) Although the measures of all our variables are acceptable in terms of conceptual and statistical criteria, improvements are especially needed for eight of the variables of our model: turnover, commitment, integration, pay, distributive justice, professionalism, general training, and kinship responsibility. The nature of these improvements will be briefly indicated for each of these variables.

Turnover should be measured as a continuous variable rather than as a dichotomy. If, for instance, twelve months elapse between measurement of the independent variables and turnover, all the stayers can be assigned scores of twelve–the maximum score. The leavers can then be assigned scores indicating the number of months they remain in the organization after completing the questionnaires; these scores will vary from one to eleven. This type of measurement of turnover might increase our explained variance since we did not differentiate the leavers in this research.

We have already indicated that commitment should be substituted for intent to stay. Fortunately, Mowday, Steers, and Porter (Mowday et al. 1979) have developed a new measure of commitment which should be used in future research.

Our present measure of integration focuses on close friends in the organization rather than in the immediate work group. It may be that it is close friends in the work group which reduces turnover; at least this possibility should be checked before integration is discarded.

We measured pay by direct monetary income. A measure of fringe benefits was developed, but too many "don't knows" were obtained for the measure to be useful. Fringe benefits are an important dimension of pay and should be measured. In addition, since pay is easily available from organizational records, it should be taken from this source rather than from questionnaires.

Our measure of distributive justice linked efforts expended to pay. This is too narrow a measure of rewards and should be expanded to include various forms of recognition, such as promotions, allocation of scarce physical resources, letters of commendation, and so forth. Distributive justice may be more important with an expanded measure of rewards.

Professionalism was measured in the traditional manner by having the nurse identify various forms of participation in professional associations. The three measures factored together and high loadings were obtained. Professionalism, however, did not turn out to be an important variable. This may be, as previously suggested, because most the nurses scored very low on our measure of professionalism. However, both nurses and some nonnursing administrators who have commented on our research have viewed our measures of professionalism in strongly negative terms. As a result of these criticisms, we now believe that more direct measures of "adherence to standards" should be used to measure professionalism. It is possible that dedication to occupational standards of performance is not indicated very well by various forms of participation in professional associations. More direct measures of dedication to occupational standards would also provide the means to study occupational groups not customarily defined as professions. Secretaries, for instance, are not viewed as professionals but differ greatly in their dedication to quality work performance.

We measured general training by type of educational training experienced by the nurses. Use of this measure is consistent with research in the human capital tradition in economics, is supported by the nurses we interviewed, and its influence was as we expected when estimated. However, this type of measure is only applicable to nurses and we prefer multiple-indicator measures. More widely applicable measures should be developed for general training. For example, it would be desirable to determine the extent to which a person's skills and knowledge are transferable to other organizations. We believe that improvement in the measurement of general training would result in it being a more important determinant.

Finally, our measure of kinship responsibility was an index based on marital status, the presence of children, and the nurse's ranking of kinship responsibilities. The element of kinship priority should be included as part of the previously discussed kinship-priority variable, and the measure of kinship responsibility should be expanded to include the presence of other relatives (parents and siblings) in the community. We were mildly surprised by how important the kinship-responsibility variable was with a barely adequate measure and are anxious to determine the effect of a better measure applied to a sample of males and females.

Further research which embodies these theoretical and procedural improvements should produce more satisfactory results. With improvements in our ability to explain variations in turnover will come the capacity to make recommendations that will significantly reduce the turnover of hospital nurses. In short, the better our causal model, the greater our power to effect intended changes.

SOME FINAL THOUGHTS ABOUT THE RESEARCH

This research has attempted to explain the turnover of hospital nurses. Explanations of this turnover should, in the long run, help hospitals render better care for their patients and exert a greater measure of control over their costs. Increased control of hospital costs should contribute to the effort to control inflation in American society, since these costs are an important component of rising prices in the society. A reduction in nursing turnover should also make the shortage of nurses less severe and make it easier to obtain a more even geographical distribution of nurses.

We have attempted to explain nursing turnover with a causal model based mostly on the research findings from studies on males who work full-time in blue-collar occupations in manufacturing industries. The most notable feature of our model is its comprehensiveness. No other model encompasses the range of determinants that we include. Inclusion of all major determinants in our model allows us to order, albeit crudely, these determinants in terms of their explanatory power. Rather than being incorporated into the model, the correlates of turnover (age and length of service) are used to check the comprehensiveness of the model and to specify similarities and differences among the nurses.

Research on the determinants of turnover has long been characterized, with a few notable exceptions, by weak analysis strategies. Intent to stay is often used as a proxy for turnover. With such a proxy, of course, data collection for the determinants occurs at the same time as data collection for the dependent variable. In short, cross-sectional designs are the rule. When turnover *per se* is measured, the leavers are often examined while the stayers are *not*. Also common to turnover research is data collection about the determinants based on verbally stated reasons for leaving, the reasons often being obtained from exit interviews conducted by the employing organization. In addition, either individuals or social systems are used as the units of analysis, but never both. Finally, and perhaps most important, there is the strong reliance on bivariate analysis; the use of statistical controls is not a pervasive characteristic of research on the determinants of turnover.

Our analysis procedures have attempted to remedy each of these weaknesses. Data about turnover were collected from interviews and records *after* data were collected about the determinants. We thus used a *longitudinal* design. Both leavers *and* stayers were studied. Hospital nurses described their situations, *and* it was the task of the analysis to see if the situations of the leavers and stayers were significantly different. The content of the situations described was, of course, prescribed by the causal model. Both individuals *and* social systems were used as the units of analysis. And finally, the *data* collected were analyzed using multiple-regression and path-analytic techniques.

Both economic and noneconomic determinants were found to be important in explaining turnover for our total sample. Also, both environmental and nonenvironmental determinants were important. In addition, we found it especially interesting that a number of determinants which we did not find to be important had been strongly supported by previous research. These conclusions were made possible because we conducted multivariate analysis with a comprehensive causal model. Of major significance are our findings for job satisfaction and intent to stay. Both are important intervening variables, and intent to stay has the largest net effect of any of the determinants. These findings for the entire sample of nurses were also basically supported when four categories of nurses were analyzed and when the nursing units were used to analyze the data—thus providing added support for our model.

It generally is assumed in most studies of the determinants of turnover that a single causal model is applicable to all categories of respondents. We, however, found differences when the model was estimated for four categories of nurses. The explanatory power of the determinants clearly varied with different categories of nurses. These findings constitute the basis for what is referred to as the contingency approach to the study of the determinants of turnover. It is important to emphasize, however, that there are numerous important similarities across the four categories, and we believe these outweigh the differences observed.

We were disappointed by our relatively low explained variance (17 percent), which was slightly less than the results indicated (23 percent) in the comprehensive review of Mobley and his colleagues (1979b).[16] We had hoped for a considerably higher explained variance, given our comprehensive causal model. Our explained variance, however, compares favorably to the 20 percent obtained in Sloan's important studies (1975; 1978: 135-165) of nursing turnover.[17]

So, though somewhat discouraged, we are still basically optimistic about our model. We are even more optimistic if future research implements the theoretical and procedural suggestions which we advanced in the preceding section. The model which we have advanced and estimated appears to provide a solid foundation for future research on the determinants of turnover.

NOTES

1. The reference here is to the total effects for these determinants.
2. As before, the reference is to total effects.
3. Following publication of the Coleman Report (Coleman et al. 1966) on educational achievements of minority-group students, a number of critics (Bowles and Levin 1968; Cain and Watts 1970; and Mosteller and Moynihan 1972) took the authors to task for using the results from regression analysis for making policy recommendations. Because a discussion of these issues would require considerable space and detailed statistical arguments, the discussion will not be presented.
4. This definition of career is based on the work of Larson (1977, p. 70).
5. The "slightly" should be emphasized since integration did not turn out to be a very important determinant in this research.
6. The crude turnover rate is also used for the hospital as the unit of analysis.
7. Material about the median length of service for leavers is found in Van der Merwe and Miller (1976, pp. 32-64) and Price (1977, pp. 11-23). Calculation of this median, obviously, will not directly reduce turnover, as will implementation of the preceding seven recommendations. As a rule, however, long-term reductions in turnover are partially the result of bet-

ter measurement. It is difficult for managers to reduce turnover unless they have adequate information produced by good measures of turnover. The median length of service of the leavers contributes to long-term reduction of turnover by providing good information about turnover.

8. These additional determinants are also discussed in Chapter 2.

9. Size here refers to the total organization—the hospital in our sample. Sometimes size refers to work units within organizations (Muchinsky and Tuttle 1979). We use size of the nursing units in Appendix 7-1. The customary pattern in the turnover literature is to use size of the organization rather than size of the work unit.

10. See Price (1972b) for a discussion of the concept of effectiveness.

11. Footnote 33 in Chapter 2 cites the literature supporting this proposition. Only one study supports coordination, another determinant cited in Chapter 2; therefore, no mention is made of coordination at this point.

12. This assumes that both males and females assign top priority to kinship roles. If only the females have this priority, as tradition prescribes, then kinship priority will result in higher turnover for females.

13. There may be an interaction between these two determinants: kinship responsibility may reduce turnover only when kinship priority is high. It is also possible that these variables operate differently for males and females. These and other questions can be settled only by further research.

14. One item from this attempted measure of kinship priority is used in the measurement of kinship responsibility. Our measurement of kinship priority by itself was not an important determinant, so it was not used in our analysis. As previously indicated, we now suggest that kinship responsibility and kinship priority are separate determinants.

15. In estimating the model we included work-unit size in Appendix 7-1.

16. The explained variance for the nursing unit is 26 percent. The explained variances when the four categories of nurses are used range from 12 percent to 26 percent.

17. Sloan's studies are very different from our research, so strict comparisons are difficult to make.

APPENDIX A
Questionnaire

STUDY OF NURSING TURNOVER

This study is conducted by Professors Myrtle K. Aydellote (College of Nursing, University of Iowa) and James L. Price (Department of Sociology, University of Iowa). The aim of the study is to learn more about why registered nurses decide to stay in or leave a hospital.

All responses to all questions are completely confidential. Completed questionnaires will be analyzed by Professors Aydelotte and Price at the University of Iowa. Findings resulting from the study will be reported statistically so that the identity of individuals and single small groups will not be revealed. None of the questionnaires, once they are filled out, will ever be seen by anyone in the hospital.

In order to study the actual leaving of nurses in the future months, it must be possible to match the questionnaire which a nurse fills out at this time with the fact that she or he either stays or leaves later. The number stamped on the top of the questionnaire makes it possible to do this matching.

INSTRUCTIONS

1. Please answer the questions in order. Do not skip around.
2. All of the questions can be answered by checking (√) one of the answers. If you do not find the exact answer that fits your case, check the one that comes closest to it. Please answer all questions.
3. Feel free to write in any explanations or comments you may have in the margins and on the back of the questionnaire.
4. Remember, the answers you give will be completely confidential. It is important that you be as honest as you can in answering this questionnaire.
5. Please return your completed questionnaire in the enclosed, prepaid envelope to Dr. Price at the University of Iowa.

ABOUT YOUR JOB

1. Are you working *full-time* or *part-time*?
( ) Full-time
( ) Part-time

2a. Do you work on a *rotating shift* or a *straight-shift*?
( ) Rotating shift
( ) Straight shift

2b. *If you work on a straight shift*, on what shift do you work?
( ) Day Shift
( ) Evening shift
( ) Night shift

3. What is the total *length of time* that you have worked in the hospital in any capacity?
( ) Less than one year
( ) Between 1-3 years
( ) Between 3-5 years
( ) Between 5-10 years
( ) Over ten years

4. How long has your *immediate supervisor* been in his or her present position? (*Note:* Your immediate supervisor is the person who *offically evaluates* your work.)
( ) Less than one year
( ) More than one year
( ) Don't know

5. What is the *official name* of the *nursing unit* on which you are now working? ______________________________
____

6. What is the total *length of time* that you have worked on the *nursing unit* on which you are now working?
( ) Less than one year
( ) Between 1-3 years
( ) Between 3-5 years
( ) Between 5-10 years
( ) Over ten years

7. How much *variety* is there in the activities that make up your job?
( ) A very great variety
( ) A great variety
( ) A moderate variety
( ) Some variety
( ) Little or no variety

8. To what extent do you do the same job in the same way every day?
( ) Almost totally the same every day
( ) Very much the same
( ) Moderately the same
( ) Somewhat the same
( ) Almost totally different every day

9. To what extent are the activities that make up your job *routine*?
( ) Very routine
( ) Quite routine
( ) Moderately routine
( ) Somewhat routine
( ) Little or no routine

10. How much *repetitiveness* is there in the activities that make up your job?
( ) A very great deal
( ) A great deal
( ) A moderate amount
( ) Some
( ) Little or none

11. Listed below are different kinds of *opportunities which a job might offer.* How much *importance* do you personally attach to each of these opportunities, disregarding whether or not your present job provides them? (Check one for each opportunity)

Opportunity	Very Important	Quite Important	Fairly Important	Somewhat Important	Not Important at All
A. To have a varied job	( )	( )	( )	( )	( )
B. To receive good pay	( )	( )	( )	( )	( )
C. To receive good fringe benefits	( )	( )	( )	( )	( )
D. To be able to get ahead	( )	( )	( )	( )	( )
E. To have close friends	( )	( )	( )	( )	( )
F. To be able to grow profes-sionally	( )	( )	( )	( )	( )
G. To be informed about your job	( )	( )	( )	( )	( )
H. To make decisions about your job	( )	( )	( )	( )	( )
I. To be fairly paid for the work you do	( )	( )	( )	( )	( )

12. How much do you *agree* or *disagree* with each of the following statements about your job? (Check one for each statement)

Statement	Strongly Agree	Agree	Neither Agree nor Disagree	Disagree	Strongly Disagree
A. I find real enjoyment in my job.	( )	( )	( )	( )	( )
B. I consider my job rather unpleasant.	( )	( )	( )	( )	( )
C. I enjoy my job more than my leisure time.	( )	( )	( )	( )	( )
D. I am often bored with my job.	( )	( )	( )	( )	( )
E. I am fairly well satis-fied with my job.	( )	( )	( )	( )	( )

Statement	Strongly Agree	Agree	Neither Agree nor Disagree	Disagree	Strongly Disagree
F. I definitely dislike my job.	( )	( )	( )	( )	( )
G. Each day on my job seems like it will never end.	( )	( )	( )	( )	( )
H. Most days I am enthusiastic about my job.	( )	( )	( )	( )	( )

PAY, FRINGE BENEFITS, AND PROMOTION

13. *Compared to the effort that you put into you job,* how do you feel about the pay you receive in the hospital?
    ( ) Compared with the effort, my pay is very poor
    ( ) Poor
    ( ) About right
    ( ) Good
    ( ) Compared with the effort, my pay is very good

14. Compared to the effort that *other nurses in the hospital* put into their jobs, how do you feel about the pay you receive in the hospital?
    ( ) Compared with the effort of other nurses, my pay is very good
    ( ) Good
    ( ) About right
    ( ) Poor
    ( ) Compared with the effort of other nurses, my pay is very poor

15. How do you feel about the pay you receive in the hospital compared to the contribution that you make toward its operation?
    ( ) Compared to my contribution, my pay is very poor
    ( ) Poor
    ( ) About right
    ( ) Good
    ( ) Compared to my contribution, my pay is very good

16. Compared to your *investment in nursing* (time, energy, experience, education, and so forth), how do you feel about the pay you receive in the hospital?
    ( ) Much more investment than pay
    ( ) More investment than pay
    ( ) Investment and pay about equal
    ( ) More pay than investment
    ( ) Much more pay than investment

17. How would you rate *your hospital* by the extent to which it makes available the following *fringe benefits* to *you*? (Check one for each fringe benefit)

Fringe Benefits	Very Good Benefits	Good Benefits	Average Benefits	Poor Benefits	Very Poor Benefits	Don't Know
A. Medical, surgical, or hospital insurance that covers any illness or injury that might occur to you while *off* the job	( )	( )	( )	( )	( )	( )
B. Life insurance that would cover a death occurring for reasons *not* connected with your job	( )	( )	( )	( )	( )	( )
C. Retirement benefits	( )	( )	( )	( )	( )	( )
D. Educational opportunities	( )	( )	( )	( )	( )	( )
E. Vacations	( )	( )	( )	( )	( )	( )
F. Sick leave	( )	( )	( )	( )	( )	( )
G. Paid holidays	( )	( )	( )	( )	( )	( )
H. Weekends off	( )	( )	( )	( )	( )	( )

18. How much do you agree or disagree with each of the following statements about *promotional opportunities* for a person with your qualifications somewhere in the hospital? (Check one for each statement)

Statement	Strongly Agree	Agree	Neither Agree nor Disagree	Disagree	Strongly Disagree
A. There is little chance to get ahead.	( )	( )	( )	( )	( )
B. Promotions are regular.	( )	( )	( )	( )	( )
C. Promotions are infrequent.	( )	( )	( )	( )	( )
D. There is an opportunity for advancement.	( )	( )	( )	( )	( )
E. I'm in a dead-end job.	( )	( )	( )	( )	( )
F. There is a very good opportunity for advancement.	( )	( )	( )	( )	( )
G. Promotions are very rare.	( )	( )	( )	( )	( )
H. There is a good chance to get ahead.	( )	( )	( )	( )	( )

CLOSE FRIENDS AT WORK

19. How many *close friends* do you have *among hospital employees*? (*Note*: There is nothing odd about having no close friends among hospital employees. Many people have close friends outside the hospital, or have no close friends.)
( ) No close friends among hospital employees
( ) One
( ) Two
( ) Three
( ) Four
( ) Five or more close friends among hospital employees

20. *While you are actually working*, how often do you see your close friends among hospital employees?
( ) More than once a day
( ) About once a day
( ) About once every two days
( ) Less than once every two days
( ) No close friends among hospital employees

21. How often do you see your close friends among hospital employees *during breaks*, such as for coffee and lunch?
( ) More than once a day
( ) About once a day
( ) About once every two days
( ) Less than once every two days
( ) No close friends among hospital employees

22. How often do you see your close friends among hospital employees *outside of working hours*, such as at dinners, picnics, or other social events?
( ) Almost every day
( ) Roughly between two and six times a week
( ) About once a week
( ) About every other week
( ) About once a month
( ) Less than once a month
( ) No close friends among hospital employees

THE JOB MARKET

23. How easy would it be for *you* to find a nursing job with another employer?
( ) Very easy
( ) Quite easy
( ) Fairly easy
( ) Not quite so easy
( ) Not easy at all

24. How easy would it be for you to find a nursing job *as good as the one you have now* with another employer?
( ) Very easy
( ) Quite easy
( ) Fairly easy
( ) Not quite so easy
( ) Not easy at all

25. How would you describe the *number of available nursing jobs*, with all types of employers, for a nurse with your qualifications?
( ) A great many
( ) Quite a few
( ) A moderate number
( ) Few
( ) Very few

26. Which of the following statements, in your view, best describes the *job market* for a nurse with your qualifications?
( ) There are more job vacancies than applicants
( ) There are more applicants than job vacancies

27. Which of the following statements most clearly reflects your feelings about your *future in the hospital?*
( ) Definitely will not leave
( ) Probably will not leave
( ) Uncertain
( ) Probably will leave
( ) Definitely will leave

COMMUNICATION AND DECISION-MAKING

28. How well *informed* are you about each of the following aspects of *your job* in the hospital? (Check one for each aspect)

Aspect	Very Well Informed	Quite Well Informed	Fairly Well Informed	Somewhat Informed	Hardly at All Informed
A. What is to be done	( )	( )	( )	( )	( )
B. Policies and procedures	( )	( )	( )	( )	( )
C. Priority of work to be done	( )	( )	( )	( )	( )
D. How well the job is done	( )	( )	( )	( )	( )
E. Technical knowledge	( )	( )	( )	( )	( )
F. Nature of equipment used	( )	( )	( )	( )	( )
G. Forthcoming changes	( )	( )	( )	( )	( )
H. How you are supposed to do the job	( )	( )	( )	( )	( )

29. Here is a list of decisions which get made on the job. For each of the following decisions, please indicate *how much say you actually have* in making these decisions. (Check one for each decision)

Decision	No Say at All	Some Say	Moderate Say	A Good Deal of Say	A Very Great Deal of Say
A. How you do your job	( )	( )	( )	( )	( )
B. Sequence of your job activities	( )	( )	( )	( )	( )

Decision	No Say at All	Some Say	Moderate Say	A Good Deal of Say	A Very Great Deal of Say
C. Speed at which you work	( )	( )	( )	( )	( )
D. Changing how you do your job	( )	( )	( )	( )	( )
E. How much you work	( )	( )	( )	( )	( )
F. When you work	( )	( )	( )	( )	( )
G. How work will be divided among people	( )	( )	( )	( )	( )
H. What you do from day to day	( )	( )	( )	( )	( )

YOUR PROFESSION

30. How many *memberships* do you have in *professional associations*, such as American Nurses' Association, Association of Operation Room Nurses, Critical Care Nurse Association, and so forth?
( ) None
( ) One
( ) Two
( ) Three
( ) Four or more

31. How many *official positions*, such as being an officer or committee member, do you have in professional associations?
( ) None
( ) One
( ) Two
( ) Three
( ) Four or more
( ) No memberships in professional associations

32. How often do you generally *attend meetings* (district, state, and national) of a professional association?
( ) Never attend meetings
( ) Between one and five times a year
( ) Between six and twelve times a year
( ) Over twelve time a year
( ) No memberships in professional associations

33. Approximately how many *nursing conferences* outside the hospital have you attended since you finished your basic education in nursing? (*Note:* Include only conferences that run two days or more)
( ) None
( ) One
( ) Two to five
( ) Six to ten
( ) Over ten

THE LOCAL COMMUNITY IN WHICH YOU LIVE

34. How many *memberships* do you have in *local community organizations*, such as churches, civic associations, fraternal orders, political groups,

trade unions, recreational clubs, and so forth?
( ) No memberships
( ) One
( ) Two
( ) Three
( ) Four
( ) Five or more memberships

35. Considering *all* of the local community organizations to which you belong, approximately how often do you generally *attend their meetings?*
( ) Less than once a week
( ) At least once a week for one organization or another
( ) Twice a week
( ) Three times a week
( ) Four times a week or more for one organization or another
( ) No memberships in local community organizations

36. How many *official positions*, such as being a committee member or an officer, do you have in these local community organizations?
( ) No official positions
( ) One
( ) Two
( ) Three
( ) Four
( ) Five or more official positions
( ) No memberships in local community organizations

37. How often do you *vote* in local community elections, such as for the school board or the city council?
( ) Vote in every election
( ) Vote in more than a majority of the elections
( ) Vote in about half of the elections
( ) Vote in less than half of the elections
( ) Never vote

ABOUT YOURSELF

Turnover is often influenced by personal characteristics such as age, education, marital status, and so forth. Therefore, some background information is needed about you.

38. How old are you?
( ) Less than 25 years old
( ) 25 to 29
( ) 30 to 34
( ) 35 to 39
( ) 40 to 49
( ) 50 to 59
( ) 60 years or over

39. How much *professional schooling in nursing* have you had?
( ) Associate degree
( ) Diploma
( ) Baccalaureate
( ) Graduate degree(s)

40. Approximately how many *miles* is it from where you live to the hospital where you work?

( ) Less than five miles
( ) Between five and fifteen miles
( ) Over fifteen miles

41. What is your present *marital* status?
( ) Married
( ) Single
( ) Widowed
( ) Divorced or separated

42. Do you have any *children?*
( ) Yes
( ) No
( ) Not applicable

43. Do you have any *preschool children?*
( ) Yes
( ) No
( ) Not applicable

44. Here are five kinds of goals admired in America today. Ideally, if you could arrange your life, which goal would you choose to emphasize most, which second most, which third, which fourth, and which least? *Assign ranks from 1 to 5, with 1 signifying "most" and 5 signifying "least."*

Rank	Goal
____	To have a successful career
____	To be a good wife (or husband)
____	To be a good mother (or a good father)
____	To be a good citizen of the community
____	To be a good member of my church or synagogue

45. How would *you* rate your *job performance* as a nurse?
( ) Much better than average
( ) Better than average
( ) About average
( ) Slightly below average
( ) Considerably below average

46. How would most of your *co-workers* rate your *job performance* as a nurse?
( ) Much better than average
( ) Better than average
( ) About average
( ) Slightly below average
( ) Considerably below average

47. How would your *immediate supervisor* rate your *job performance* as a nurse?
( ) Much better than average
( ) Better than average
( ) About average'
( ) Slightly below average
( ) Considerably below average

48. While you were growing up, say until you were eighteen, what kind of community did you live in for the most part?
( ) Rural area or farm
( ) Town or small city (under 50,000)

( ) Medium-size city (50,000-250,000)
( ) Suburban area near large city
( ) Large city (over 250,000)

49. What is the *primary occupation* of your husband (or wife)?
( ) Salaried manager or official
( ) Owner of a business
( ) Clerical and kindred worker (white collar)
( ) Sales worker
( ) Professional and/or technical person (such as a doctor or engineer)
( ) Skilled craftsman (such as a carpenter) or foreman
( ) Semi-skilled worker (such as a truck driver)
( ) Laborer
( ) Private household worker (such as a maid or gardener)
( ) Other service worker (such as a waiter or waitress)
( ) Farmer or farm manager
( ) Farm laborer or foreman
( ) No present occupation (such as housewife or student)
( ) Not applicable (single, widowed, divorced or separated)

50. Do you expect to *leave the hospital* in the near future?
( ) Will definitely leave in the near future
( ) The chances are quite good that I will leave
( ) The situation is uncertain
( ) The chances are very slight that I will leave
( ) Definitely will not leave in the near future

Note: The two following questions on income are *very important* because many people beleive that income is a significant factor in explaining nursing turnover. Like all the other information collected by this questionnaire, the information about income is completely confidential.

51. *Roughly*, what is *your* total yearly income from nursing before taxes and other deductions are made?
( ) Less than $3,000
( ) $3,000 to $4,999
( ) $5,000 to $6,999
( ) $7,000 to $8,999
( ) $9,000 to $10,000
( ) $11,000 to $12,999
( ) $13,000 to $14,999
( ) $15,000 or over

52. *Roughly*, what is the total yearly income before taxes and other deductions of *your immediate family*-including your own income, the income of everyone else in the family who works, and income from any other source?
( ) Less than $5,000
( ) $5,000 to $7,499
( ) $7,500 to $9,999
( ) $10,000 to $12,499
( ) $12,500 to $14,999
( ) $15,000 to $19,999
( ) $20,000 to $24,999
( ) $25,000 to $29,999
( ) $30,000 or over
( ) Not applicable (I am single income-earner)

PLEASE CHECK TO MAKE SURE YOU HAVEN'T SKIPPED ANY QUESTIONS

Thank you very much for your cooperation in filling out this questionnaire.

If you have any further ideas or comments you would like to make, please feel free to use the bottom and back of this page to write them on.

APPENDIX B
Measurement

INTENT TO STAY

27. Which of the following statements most clearly reflects your feelings about your *future in the hospital?*

	Score
( ) Definitely will not leave	4
( ) Probably will not leave	3
( ) Uncertain	2
( ) Probably will leave	1
( ) Definitely will leave	0

50. Do you expect to *leave the hospital* in the near future?

	Score
( ) Will definitely leave in the near future	0
( ) The chances are quite good that I will leave	1
( ) The situation is uncertain	2
( ) The chances are very slight that I will leave	3
( ) Definitely will not leave in the near future	4

Notes: The score for intent to stay is obtained by summing the scores for the two items. The same practice is followed for the other indices.

12. How much do you *agree* or *disagree* with each of the following statements about your job? (Check one for each statement)

Statement	Strongly Agree	Agree	Neither Agree nor Disagree	Disagree	Strongly Disagree
A. I find real enjoyment in my job	( )	( )	( )	( )	( )
B. I consider my job rather unpleasant.	( )	( )	( )	( )	( )
D. I am often bored with my job.	( )	( )	( )	( )	( )
E. I am fairly well satisfied with my job.	( )	( )	( )	( )	( )

Statement	Strongly Agree	Agree	Neither Agree nor Disagree	Disagree	Strongly Disagree
F. I definitely dislike my job.	( )	( )	( )	( )	( )
G. Each day on my job seems like it will never end.	( )	( )	( )	( )	( )
H. Most days I am enthusiastic about my job.	( )	( )	( )	( )	( )

Notes: The scoring for statements A, E, and H are as follows: Strongly Agree = four; Agree = three; Neither Agree nor Disagree = two; Disagree = one; and Strongly Disagree = zero. The scoring is reversed for statements B, D, F, and G. One statement (C), whose loading was .41, was dropped as a result of the factor analysis. A single factor was obtained, whose loadings for statement A through H are, respectively, .78, .70, .61, .69, .76, .62, and .74.

OPPORTUNITY

23. How easy would it be for *you* to find a nursing job with another employer?

	Score
( ) Very easy	4
( ) Quite easy	3
( ) Fairly easy	2
( ) Not quite so easy	1
( ) Not easy at all	0

24. How easy would it be for you to find a nursing job *as good as the one you now have* with another employer?

	Score
( ) Very easy	4
( ) Quite easy	3
( ) Fairly easy	2
( ) Not quite so easy	1
( ) Not easy at all	0

25. How would you describe the *number of available nursing jobs*, with all types of employers, for a nurse with your qualifications?

	Score
( ) A great many	4
( ) Quite a few	3
( ) A moderate number	2
( ) Few	1
( ) Very few	0

26. Which of the following statements, in your view, best describes the *job market* for a nurse with your qualifications?

	Score
( ) There are more job vacancies than applicants	1
( ) There are more applicants than job vacancies	0

Notes: The factor analysis yielded a single factor. The factor loadings on Questions 23-26 are, respectively, as follows: .70, .63, .65, and .53.

ROUTINIZATION

7. How much *variety* is there in the activities that make up your job?

	Score
( ) A very great variety	0
( ) A great variety	1
( ) A moderate variety	2
( ) Some variety	3
( ) Little or no variety	4

8. To what extent do you do the same job in the same way every day?

	Score
( ) Almost totally the same every day	4
( ) Very much the same	3
( ) Moderately the same	2
( ) Somewhat the same	1
( ) Almost totally different every day	0

9. To what extent are the activities that make up your job *routine*?

	Score
( ) Very routine	4
( ) Quite routine	3
( ) Moderately routine	2
( ) Somewhat routine	1
( ) Little or no routine	0

10. How much *repetitiveness* is there in the activities that make up your job?

	Score
( ) A very great deal	4
( ) A great deal	3
( ) A moderate amount	2
( ) Some	1
( ) Little or none	0

Notes: The factor analysis yielded a single factor. The factor loadings on Questions 7-10 are, respectively, as follows: .60, .72, .77, and .73.

PARTICIPATION

29. Here is a list of decisions which get made on the job. For each of the following decisions, please indicate *how much say you actually have* in making these decisions. (Check one for each decision)

Decision	No Say at All	Some Say	Moderate Say	A Good Deal of Say	A Very Great Deal of Say
A. How you do your job	( )	( )	( )	( )	( )
B. Sequence of your job activities	( )	( )	( )	( )	( )
C. Speed at which you work	( )	( )	( )	( )	( )
D. Changing how you do your job	( )	( )	( )	( )	( )

Notes: The scoring for the responses is as follows: No Say at All = four; Some Say = three; Moderate Say = two; A Good Deal of Say = one;

and A Very Great Deal of Say = zero. The factor loadings for decisions A-D are, respectively, as follows: .74, .77, .73, and .66. The original questionnaire also had four more decisions, E-H; the loadings on these items are .42, .21, .25, and .28. Two factors were obtained in the factor analysis and only the above items were used to represent participation. (The loadings for decisions A-H for the excluded second factor are as follows: .26, .30, .28, .35, .39, .42, .70, and .78.)

INSTRUMENTAL COMMUNICATION

28. How well *informed* are you about each of the following aspects of *your job* in the hospital? (Check one for each aspect)

Aspects	Very Well Informed	Quite Well Informed	Fairly Well Informed	Somewhat Informed	Hardly at All Informed
A. What is to be done	( )	( )	( )	( )	( )
B. Policies and procedures	( )	( )	( )	( )	( )
C. Priority of work to be done	( )	( )	( )	( )	( )
D. How well the job is done	( )	( )	( )	( )	( )
E. Technical knowledge	( )	( )	( )	( )	( )
F. Nature of equipment used	( )	( )	( )	( )	( )
H. How you are supposed to do the job	( )	( )	( )	( )	( )

Notes: The scoring for the aspects is as follows: Very Well Informed = four; Quite Well Informed = three; Fairly Well Informed = two; Somewhat Informed = one; and Hardly at All Informed = zero. A single factor was obtained. The factor loadings for aspects A-H are, respectively, as follows: .75, .71, .77, .72, .75, .73, and .78. One aspect (G) was excluded because of a small loading (.53).

INTEGRATION

19. How many *close friends* do you have among *hospital employees? (Note:* There is nothing odd about having no close friends among hospital employees. Many people have close friends outside the hospital, or have no close friends.)

	Score
( ) No close friends among hospital employees	0
( ) One	1
( ) Two	2
( ) Three	3
( ) Four	4
( ) Five or more close friends among hospital employees	5

20. *While you are actually working,* how often do you see your close friends among hospital employees?

	Score
( ) More than once a day	4
( ) About once a day	3

	Score
( ) About once every two days	2
( ) Less than once every two days	1
( ) No close friends among hospital employees	9

21. How often do you see your close friends among hospital employees *during breaks*, such as for coffee and lunch?

	Score
( ) More than once a day	4
( ) About once a day	3
( ) About once every two days	2
( ) Less than once every two days	1
( ) No close friends among hospital employees	9

22. How often do you see your close friends among hospital employees *outside of working hours*, such as at dinners, picnics, or other social events?

	Score
( ) Almost every day	6
( ) Roughly between two and six times a week	5
( ) About once a week	4
( ) About every other week	3
( ) About once a month	2
( ) Less than once a month	1
( ) No close friends among hospital employees	9

Notes: A single factor was obtained in the factor analysis. The loadings for Questions 19-22 are, respectively, as follows: .65, .85, .84, and .58.

PAY

51. *Roughly*, what is *your* total yearly income from nursing before taxes and other deductions are made:

	Score
( ) Less than $3,000	$ 1,500
( ) $3,000 to $4,999	$ 4,000
( ) $5,000 to $6,999	$ 6,000
( ) $7,000 to $8,999	$ 8,000
( ) $9,000 to $10,999	$ 10,000
( ) $11,000 to $12,999	$ 12,000
( ) $13,000 to $14,999	$ 14,000
( ) $15,000 or over	$ 16,000

DISTRIBUTIVE JUSTICE

13. *Compared to the effort that you put into your job,* how do you feel about the pay you receive in the hospital?

	Score
( ) Compared with the effort, my pay is very poor	0
( ) Poor	1
( ) About right	2
( ) Good	1
( ) Compared with the effort, my pay is very good	0

14. Compared to the effort that *other nurses in the hospital* put into their jobs, how do you feel about the pay you receive in the hospital?

	Score
( ) Compared with the effort of other nurses, my pay is good	0

	Score
( ) Good	1
( ) About right	2
( ) Poor	1
( ) Compared with the effort of other nurses, my pay is very poor	0

15. How do you feel about the pay you receive in the hospital compared to the contribution that you make toward its operation?

	Score
( ) Compared to my contribution, my pay is very poor	0
( ) Poor	1
( ) About right	2
( ) Good	1
( ) Compared to my contribution, my pay is very good	0

Notes: A single factor was obtained in the factor analysis. The loadings for Questions 13-15 are, respectively, as follows: .71, .62, and .71. Question 16 was eliminated because of a low loading (.39).

PROMOTIONAL OPPORTUNITY

18. How much do you agree or disagree with each of the following statements about *promotional opportunities* for a person with your qualifications somewhere in the hospital? (Check one for each statement)

Statement	Strongly Agree	Agree	Neither Agree nor Disagree	Disagree	Strongly Disagree
A. There is little chance to get ahead.	( )	( )	( )	( )	( )
B. Promotions are regular.	( )	( )	( )	( )	( )
C. Promotions are infrequent.	( )	( )	( )	( )	( )
D. There is an opportunity for advancement.	( )	( )	( )	( )	( )
E. I'm in a dead-end job.	( )	( )	( )	( )	( )
F. There is a very good opportunity for advancement.	( )	( )	( )	( )	( )
G. Promotions are very rare.	( )	( )	( )	( )	( )
H. There is a good chance to get ahead.	( )	( )	( )	( )	( )

Notes: The scoring for statements A, C, E, and G is as follows: Strongly Agree = zero; Agree = one; Neither Agree nor Disagree = two; Disagree = three; and Strongly Disagree = four. This scoring is reversed for statements B, D, F, and H. A single factor was obtained for the eight statements. The factor loadings for statements A-H are, respectively, .81, .74, .75, .75, .69, .83, .79, and .89.

PROFESSIONALISM

30. How many *memberships* do you have in *professional associations*, such as American Nurses' Association, Association of Operating Room

Nurses, Critical Care Nurse Association, and so forth?

	Score
( ) None	0
( ) One	1
( ) Two	2
( ) Three	3
( ) Four or more	4

31. How many *offical positions*, such as being an officer or committee member, do you have in professional associations?

	Score
( ) None	0
( ) One	1
( ) Two	2
( ) Three	3
( ) Four or more	4
( ) No membership in professional associations	9

32. How often do you generally *attend meetings* (district, state, and national) of a professional association?

	Score
( ) Never attend meetings	1
( ) Between one and five times a year	2
( ) Between six and twelve times a year	3
( ) Over twelve times a year	4
( ) No memberships in professional associations	9

Notes: A single factor was obtained in the factor analysis. The factor loadings for Questions 30-32 are, respectively, .72, .54, and .73. Question 33 was dropped because of a low loading (.37).

GENERAL TRAINING

39. How much *professional schooling in nursing* have you had?

	Score
( ) Associate	2
( ) Diploma	1
( ) Baccalaureate	3
( ) Graduate degree(s)	3

KINSHIP RESPONSIBILITY

41. What is your present *marital* status?
( ) Married
( ) Single
( ) Widowed
( ) Divorced or separated

42. Do you have any children?
( ) Yes
( ) No
( ) Not applicable

44. Here are five kinds of goals admired in America today. Ideally, if you could arrange your life, which goal would you choose to emphasize most, which second most, which third, which fourth, and which least? *Assign ranks from 1 to 5, with 1 signifying "most" and 5 signifying "least."*

Rank	Goal
____	To have a successful career
____	To be a good wife (or husband)
____	To be a good mother (or a good father)
____	To be a good citizen of the community
____	To be a good member of my church or synagogue

Notes:

Combinations for Questions 41, 42, and 44	Score
Not married, no children, and both good wife and good mother ranked three or lower	2
Not married, no children, and either good wife or good mother ranked two or higher	3
Not married with children or married with no children and good wife or good mother ranked three or lower	3
Not married, no children, and both good wife and good mother ranked two or higher	4
Not married with children or married with no children and either good wife or good mother ranked two or higher	4
Married with children and both good wife and good mother ranked three or lower	4
Married with children and either good wife or good mother ranked two or higher	5
Not married with children or married with no children and both good wife and good mother ranked two or higher	5
Married with children and both good wife and good mother ranked two or higher	6

AGE

38. How old are you?

	Score
( ) Less than 25 year old	0
( ) 25 to 29	0
( ) 30 to 34	1
( ) 35 to 39	1
( ) 40 to 49	1
( ) 50 to 59	1
( ) 60 years or over	1

Notes: Zero equals "young" and one equals "old."

LENGTH OF SERVICE

3. What is the total *length of time* you have worked in the hospital in any capacity?

	Score
( ) Less than one year	1
( ) Between 1-3 years	2
( ) Between 3-5 years	3
( ) Between 5-10 years	4
( ) Over ten years	5

APPENDIX C

Correlation Matrices for the Four Categories of Nurses

Table 1: Correlation Matrix for Full-Time Under Thirty[a]

	1	2	3	4	5	6	7	8	9	10	11	12	13	14	15	16
1.	--															
2.	-.371	--														
3.	-.043	.213	--													
4.	.205	-.113	.076	--												
5.	-.035	-.057	-.388	-.067	--											
6.	-.032	.148	.231	.144	-.120	--										
7.	.049	.133	.229	-.002	-.133	.324	--									
8.	-.083	.149	.099	-.046	-.105	.073	.152	--								
9.	.032	.042	.010	.046	.076	.088	.095	.047	--							
10.	-.045	.109	.088	.023	-.039	.002	.069	.005	.096	--						
11.	-.024	.168	.242	.115	-.178	.158	.143	-.009	-.042	.230	--					
12.	.009	.078	.022	.006	-.112	-.004	.039	.140	.070	-.018	.016	--				
13.	.190	-.276	.090	.239	-.048	.014	-.098	-.185	.007	-.043	.038	-.025	--			
14.	-.031	.092	-.027	-.114	.056	.006	-.011	-.117	.026	-.059	-.031	-.056	-.203	--		
15.	-.034	.129	-.076	-.120	-.052	.052	.012	.048	.202	-.070	-.143	.073	-.098	.203	--	
16.	-.121	.249	-.044	-.167	-.086	.022	.062	.230	.137	-.037	-.172	.057	-.254	.131	.399	--
x	.24	5.84	27.66	11.81	11.97	13.83	29.95	9.93	$10157	6.95	21.76	1.82	1.66	4.03	23.73	2.38
SD	.43	1.94	3.92	2.58	2.86	3.35	4.91	5.35	$ 1526	1.58	5.77	1.37	.85	1.32	2.38	.92

[a]Pairwise N's used to compute the correlations range from 434 to 467.

Note: 1 = Turnover, 2 = Intent to Stay, 3 - Job Satisfaction, 4 = Opportunity, 5 = Routinization, 6 = Participation, 7 = Instrumental Communication, 8 = Integration, 9 = Pay, 10 = Distributive Justice, 11 = Promotional Opportunity, 12 = Professionalism, 13 = General Training, 14 = Kinship Responsibility, 15 = Age, 16 = Length of Service.

Table 2: Correlation Matrix for Full-Time Thirty and Over[a]

	1	2	3	4	5	6	7	8	9	10	11	12	13	14	15	16
1.	--															
2.	-.457	--														
3.	-.198	.368	--													
4.	.027	-.155	-.210	--												
5.	-.013	-.021	-.492	.011	--											
6.	-.133	.154	.238	.162	-.075	--										
7.	.014	.063	.283	.116	-.182	.345	--									
8.	.013	.187	.187	-.120	-.094	.150	.146	--								
9.	-.103	.253	.133	-.132	-.076	-.006	.000	-.014	--							
10.	.058	-.076	.062	-.147	-.076	-.155	-.110	.103	.023	--						
11.	-.041	.107	.316	-.040	-.223	.122	.145	.198	.072	.125	--					
12.	.079	-.090	.020	.047	-.251	-.025	.074	.026	.106	-.043	.016	--				
13.	-.011	-.072	.114	.018	-.091	.041	-.053	.027	-.051	.029	.007	-.054	--			
14.	-.056	.176	.187	.053	.060	.062	.040	.078	-.056	.055	.073	-.108	-.059	--		
15.	-.116	.204	.075	-.129	.094	-.002	.067	.052	.083	.038	.014	.024	-.034	.072	--	
16.	-.101	.286	-.024	-.197	.076	.138	.184	.122	.202	.048	-.079	-.004	-.275	.024	.300	--
x	.08	7.35	28.45	10.94	12.19	14.01	27.53	7.67	$10644	6.79	21.06	2.08	1.26	5.31	44.32	4.04
SD	.28	1.94	4.72	2.78	3.05	3.86	5.33	5.02	$ 1546	1.74	6.45	1.53	.61	1.04	8.76	1.20

[a]Pairwise N's used to compute the correlations range from 185 to 203.

Note: 1 = Turnover, 2 = Intent to Stay, 3 = Job Satisfaction, 4 = Opportunity, 5 = Routinization, 6 = Participation, 7 = Instrumental Communication, 8 = Integration, 9 = Pay, 10 = Distributive Justice, 11 = Promotional Opportunity, 12 = Professionalism, 13 = General Training, 14 = Kinship Responsibility, 15 = Age, 16 = Length of Service.

Table 3: Correlation Matrix for Part-Time Under Thirty[a]

	1	2	3	4	5	6	7	8	9	10	11	12	13	14	15	16
1.	--															
2.	-.399	--														
3.	-.283	.306	--													
4.	.310	-.243	-.027	--												
5.	.146	-.093	-.327	.059	--											
6.	-.008	.116	.331	.051	-.196	--										
7.	-.231	.058	.218	.131	-.104	.273	--									
8.	.037	-.052	.038	.066	-.008	.009	.034	--								
9.	.041	-.236	-.186	.148	.075	.002	.156	.111	--							
10.	-.003	.033	-.031	-.053	.020	-.011	-.058	-.061	-.001	--						
11.	-.095	.053	.235	.081	-.153	.194	.073	-.087	-.119	.148	--					
12.	.008	.001	.141	.051	-.110	.074	.046	.093	.167	-.119	-.069	--				
13.	.208	-.127	.035	.211	.041	.120	-.040	.008	.126	-.014	.027	.021	--			
14.	-.167	.396	.128	-.200	-.095	.022	-.082	-.043	-.299	.019	-.037	.012	-.344	--		
15.	-.144	.085	.139	-.114	-.107	-.148	.066	-.138	-.168	.089	-.104	-.016	-.293	.185	--	
16.	-.294	.214	.018	-.256	-.038	-.080	.147	.081	-.052	-.090	-.148	.070	-.268	.184	.414	--
x	.30	6.05	28.34	11.46	11.85	13.81	25.71	8.17	$5849	7.24	21.29	1.60	1.47	5.52	25.45	2.77
SD	.46	2.07	3.71	2.68	2.98	3.17	4.90	4.99	$2404	1.57	5.78	1.29	.73	1.03	2.32	.98

[a]Pairwise N's used to compute the correlations range from 161 to 171.

Note: 1 = Turnover, 2 = Intent to Stay, 3 = Job Satisfaction, 4 = Opportunity, 5 = Routinization, 6 = Participation, 7 = Instrumental Communication, 8 = Integration, 9 = Pay, 10 = Distributive Justice, 11 = Promotional Opportunity, 12 = Professionalism, 13 = General Training, 14 = Kinship Responsibility, 15 = Age, 16 = Length of Service.

Table 4: Correlation Matrix for Part-Time Thirty and Over[a]

	1	2	3	4	5	6	7	8	9	10	11	12	13	14	15	16
1.	--															
2.	-.312	--														
3.	-.002	.331	--													
4.	.043	-.079	.053	--												
5.	-.009	-.128	-.262	-.103	--											
6.	-.021	.022	.225	.170	-.168	--										
7.	.067	.168	.465	.156	-.037	.295	--									
8.	-.114	.065	.055	.040	-.053	.083	.078	--								
9.	.035	.145	.182	-.035	-.024	-.015	.180	.073	--							
10.	-.113	.087	.017	-.003	-.017	-.022	.040	.011	-.019	--						
11.	.087	.058	.281	.154	.178	.184	.127	.013	-.062	.085	--					
12.	-.052	-.023	-.121	.201	-.062	.040	.041	.194	.024	-.118	-.073	--				
13.	-.003	-.180	-.225	.038	.068	-.169	-.052	-.080	.053	-.013	-.016	.045	--			
14.	-.110	-.049	-.057	.022	-.076	-.065	-.065	.065	-.080	.099	-.102	-.042	-.123	--		
15.	-.016	-.036	.070	-.102	.183	.051	.123	-.030	.090	-.064	.076	-.020	.012	-.225	--	
16.	-.133	.212	.089	-.121	-.013	.067	.121	.128	.052	.086	.058	-.090	-.216	.074	.224	--
x	.11	6.88	29.25	10.95	11.74	13.94	26.72	6.71	$5113	7.15	22.11	1.61	1.19	5.68	40.26	3.90
SD	.31	1.92	3.60	2.73	2.91	3.53	4.84	4.85	$2273	1.65	6.40	1.17	.54	.76	8.39	1.22

[a]Pairwise N's used to compute the correlations range from 218 to 243.

Note: 1 = Turnover, 2 = Intent to Stay, 3 = Job Satisfaction, 4 = Opportunity, 5 = Routinization, 6 = Participation, 7 = Instrumental Communication, 8 = Integration, 9 = Pay, 10 = Distributive Justice, 11 = Promotional Opportunity, 12 = Professionalism, 13 = General Training, 14 = Kinship Responsibility, 15 = Age, 16 = Length of Service.

References

Aitken, Hugh G. J. 1960. Taylorism at Watertown Arsenal (Cambridge, Ma.: Harvard Univ. Press).

Albrow, Martin. 1970. Bureaucracy (New York: Praeger).

Aldrich, Howard E. 1979. Organizations and Environments (Englewood Cliffs, N.J.: Prentice-Hall).

Alexander, Karl L., and Bruce K. Eckland. 1977. High school context and college selectivity: Institutional constraints in educational stratification, Social Forces 56: 166-188.

Allison, Paul D. 1978. Measures of inequality, Am. Sociol. Rev. 43:865-880.

Altman, Stuart H. 1972. Present & Future Supply of Registered Nurses (Bethesda, Md.: U.S. Department of Health, Education, and Welfare, Publication No. (NIH) 73-134).

Alwin, Duane F. 1974. College effects on educational and occupational attainments. Am. Sociol. Rev. 39:210-223.

American Hospital Association. 1977. Guide to the Health Care Field (Chicago: American Hospital Association).

American Nurses' Association. 1954. Spot Check of Nursing in Non-Federal General Hospitals (Kansas City: Research and Statistics Unit, American Nurses' Association).

———. 1962. Spot Check of Current Hospital Employment Conditions (Kansas City: Research and Statistics Unit, American Nurses' Association).

Anderson, Odin W. 1968. Toward an Unambiguous Profession? A Review of Nursing (Chicago: Center for Health Administration Studies, Graduate School of Business, Univ. of Chicago, Health Administration Perspectives No. A6).

Anderson, Peggy. 1978. Nurse (New York: St. Martin's Press).

Archibald, Kathleen A. 1971. The Supply of Professional Nurses and Their Recruitment and Retention by Hospitals (New York: Rand Institute).

Argyris, Chris. 1960. Understanding Organizational Behavior (Homewood, Ill.: Dorsey).

———. 1973. Personality and organization theory revisited, Admin. Sci. Quart. 18:141-167.

Atchison, T.J., and E.A. Lefferts. 1972. The prediction of turnover using Herzberg's job satisfaction technique, Personnel Psychol. 25:53-64.
Baldamus, W. 1951. Type of work and motivation, Brit. J. Sociol. 2:44-58.
Beattie, Christopher, and Byron G. Spencer. 1971. Career attainment in Canadian bureaucracies: Unscrambling the effects of age, seniority, education, and ethnolinguistic factors on salary, Am. J. Sociol. 77:472-490.
Becker, Gary S. 1962. Investment in human capital: A theoretical analysis, J. Political Econ. 70:9-49.
———. 1964. Human Capital (New York: Columbia Univ. Press).
Becker, Selwyn W., and Duncan Neuhauser. 1975. The Efficient Organization (New York: Elsevier).
Bell, Daniel. 1973. The Coming of Post-Industrial Society (New York: Basic Books).
Blalock, Hubert M., Jr. 1967. Path coefficients versus regression coefficients, Am. J. Sociol. 72:675-676.
Blau, Peter M. 1959-1960. Social integration, social rank, and processes of interaction, Human Organization 18:152-157.
———. 1960a. A theory of social integration, Am. J. Sociol. 65:545-556.
———. 1960b. Structural effects, Am. Sociol. Rev. 25:178-193.
———. 1973. The Organization of Academic Work (New York: Wiley).
———. 1974. Recruiting faculty and students, Sociol. Ed. 47:93-113.
Bluedorn, Allen C. 1976. A causal model of turnover in organizations (unpublished Ph.D. dissertation, Univ. of Iowa).
———. 1978. A taxonomy of turnover, Acad. Management Rev. 3:647-651.
Bohrnstedt, George W. 1970. Reliability and validity assessment in attitude measurement, Attitude Measurement, ed. G.F. Summers (Chicago: Rand McNally).
Bowey, Angela M. 1974. A Guide to Manpower Planning (London: Macmillan).
Bowles, S., and H. Levin. 1968. More on multicollinearity and the effectiveness of schools, J. Human Resources 3:393-400.
Brief, A.P. 1976. Turnover among hospital nurses: A suggested model, J. Nursing Admin. 6:55-58.
Brief, A.P., and Ramon J. Aldag. 1977. Antecedents of Organizational Commitment Among Hospital Nurses (Iowa City: Bureau of Business and Economic Research, College of Business Administration, Univ. of Iowa, Working Paper Ser. NO. 77-23).
Burns, T. 1954. The directions of activity and communication in a department executive group: A quantitative study in a British engineering factory with a self-recording technique, Human Relations 7:73-97.
Burton, John F., and John E. Parker. 1969. Interindustry variations in voluntary labor mobility, Ind. Labor Relations Rev. 22:199-216.
Cain, G.C., and H.W. Watts. 1970. Problems in making policy inferences from the Coleman report, Am. Sociol. Rev. 35:228-242.
Campbell, D.T., and D.W. Fiske. 1959. Convergent and discriminant validation by the multitrait-multimethod matrix, Psychological Bull. 56:81-105.
Caplow, Theodore, and Reece J. McGee. 1958. The Academic Marketplace (New York: Basic Books).
Carlson, Richard O. 1962. Executive Succession and Organizational Change (Chicago: Midwest Administration Center, Univ. of Chicago).
Carrell, Michael R., and John E. Dittrich. 1978. Equity theory: The recent literature, methodological considerations, and new directions, Acad. Management Rev. 3:202-210.

Charters, W.W. 1954. The effects of school district reorganization upon teacher turnover in Illinois high schools (unpublished, Bureau of Educational Research, Univ. of Illinois).

Cohen, Jacob, and Patricia Cohen. 1975. Applied Multiple Regressional Correlation Analysis for the Behavioral Sciences (Hillsdale, N.J.: Lawrence Erlbaum).

Cole, Robert E. 1971. Japanese Blue Collar (Berkeley: Univ. California Press).

Coleman, J.S., E.Q. Campbell, C.F. Hobson, J. McPartland, A.M. Mood. 1966. Equality of Educational Opportunity (Washington, D.C.: U.S. Office of Education).

Comay, Yochanan. 1972. The migration of professionals: An empirical analysis, Can. J. Econ. 5:419-429.

Corwin, Ronald G. 1961. Role conception and career aspiration: A study of identity in nursing, Sociological Quart. 2:69-86.

Cronbach, L.J. 1951. Coefficient alpha and the internal structure of tests, Psychometrika 16:297-334.

Dalton, Dan R., and William D. Tudor. 1979. Turnover turned over: An expanded and positive perspective, Acad. Management Rev. 4:225-235.

Davis, Fred (ed.). 1966. The Nursing Profession: Five Sociological Essays (New York: Wiley).

Duncan, Otis Dudley. 1966. Path analysis: Sociological examples, Am. J. Sociol. 72:1-16.

Eaton, Fred R. 1968. A study of factors which influence registered staff nurses to remain in the employment of a metropolitan teaching hospital (unpublished, Program in Hospital Administration, Univ. of Minnesota).

Eitzen, D. Stanley, and Normal R. Yetman. 1972. Managerial change, longevity, and organizational effectiveness, Admin. Sci. Quart. 17:110-116.

Fabricant, Solomon. 1969. A Primer on Productivity (New York: Random House).

Fainsod, Merle. 1963. How Russia Is Ruled (Cambridge: Harvard University Press).

Farrell, Dan. 1978. A causal model of job satisfaction (unpublished Ph.D. dissertation, Univ. of Iowa).

Farris, George F. 1971. A predictive study of turnover, Personnel Psychol. 24:311-328.

Firebaugh, G. 1978. A rule for inferring individual-level relationships from aggregate data, Am. Sociol. Rev. 43:557-572.

Flango, Victor E., and Robert B. Brumbaugh. 1974. The dimensionality of the cosmopolitan-local construct, Admin. Sci. Quart. 19:198-210.

Freidson, Eliot. 1971. Profession of Medicine, A Study of the Sociology of Applied Knowledge (New York: Dodd, Mead).

Fry, Fred L. 1973. A behavioral analysis of economic variables affecting turnover, J. Behav. Econ. 2:247-295.

Fuchs, Victor R. 1968. The Service Economy (New York: National Bureau of Economic Research, No. 87, Gen. Ser.).

Galbraith, Jay. 1973. Designing Complex Organizations (Reading, Ma.: Addison-Wesley).

Gannon, Martin J., and Joseph C. Nothern. 1971. A comparison of short-term and long-term part-time employees, Personnel Psychol. 24:687-696.

__________, and Uri Brainin. 1971. Employee tenure in the temporary help industry, Industrial Relations 10: 168-175.

Gillespie, Michael W. 1977. Log-linear techniques and the regression analysis of dummy dependent variables: Further bases for comparison, Sociol. Methods Res. 6:103-122.

Goode, Williams J. 1960. Encroachment, charlatanism, and the emerging profession, Am. Sociol. Rev. 25:902-914.
Goodman, Leo A. 1976. The relationship between the modified and more usual multiple regression approaches to the analysis of dichotomous variables, Sociological Methodology, ed. David R. Heise (San Francisco: Jossey-Bass).
Goodman, Paul S., Paul Salipante, and Harold Paransky. 1973. Hiring, training, and retaining the hardcore unemployed: A selected review, J. Appl. Psychol. 58:23-33.
Gordon, Robert A. 1968. Issues in multiple regression, Am. J. Sociol. 73:592-616.
Gouldner, Alvin W. 1957. Cosmopolitans and locals. Toward an analysis of latent social roles—I, Admin. Sci. Quart. 2:281-306.
————. 1958. Cosmopolitans and locals. Toward an analysis of latent social roles—II, Admin. Sci. Quart. 2:444-480.
Gowler, Dan. 1969. Determinants of the supply of labor to the firm, J. Management Studies 6:73-95.
Greeley, Andrew M. 1972. Priests in the United States (Garden City, N.J.: Doubleday).
Grusky, Oscar. 1960. Administrative succession in formal organizations, Social Forces 39:21-31.
————. 1964. The effects of succession: A comparative study of military and business organization, The New Military, ed. Morris Janowtiz (New York: Russell Sage Foundation).
Hauser, Robert M. 1972. Socioeconomic Background and Educational Performance (Washington, D.C.: American Sociological Association).
Heberlein, Thomas A., and Robert Baumgartner. 1978. Factors affecting response rates to mailed questionnaires: A quantitative analysis of the published literature, Am. Sociol. Rev. 43:447-462.
Heise, D.R. 1972. Employing nominal variables, induced variables, and block variables in path analysis, Sociological Methods and Research 1: 147-173.
Herzberg, Frederick, Bernard Mausner, Richard O. Peterson, and Dora F. Capwell. 1957. Job Attitudes (Pittsburgh: Psychological Service of Pittsburgh).
Hill, J.M.M. 1952. Approach to labor turnover. The Engineer 194:306-309.
Hinrichs, J.R. 1971. The exit interview, Personnel 48:30-35.
————. 1975. Measurement of reasons for resignation of professionals: Questionnaire versus company and consultant exit interviews, J. Appl. Psychol. 60:530-532.
Hirschman, Albert O. 1970. Exit, Voice and Loyalty (Cambridge, Ma.: Harvard Univ. Press).
Homans, George Caspar. 1961. Social Behavior - Its Elementary Forms (New York: Harcourt, Brace).
————. 1967. The Nature of Social Science (New York: Harcourt, Brace).
Hughes, Everett, Helen MacGill Hughes, Erwin Deutscher, 1958. Twenty Thousand Nurses Tell Their Story (Philadelphia: Lippincott).
Hunter, J.A. 1962. Turnover among beginning teachers - A followup, School Life 44:22-24.
Ingham, Geoffrey K. 1967. Organization size, orientation to work and industrial relations, Sociol. 1:239-258.
————. 1970. Size of Industrial Organization and Worker Behavior (Cambridge, Eng.: Cambridge Univ. Press).
Johnson, Harry M. 1960. Sociology (New York: Harcourt).
Jöreskog, Karl G. 1970. A general method for estimating a linear struc-

tural equation system, Structural Equation Models in the Social Sciences, eds. A.S. Goldberger and O.D. Duncan (New York: Seminar Press).
________, and Dag Sorböm. 1978. Lisrel User's Guide (Uppsala, Swed.: Univ. of Uppsala).
Kanungo, Rabindra N. 1979. The concepts of alienation and involvement revisisted. Psychological Bull. 86:119-138.
Katz, Ralph. 1978. Job longevity as a situational factor in job satisfaction, Admin. Sci. Quart. 23:204-223.
Kendrick, John W. 1977. Understanding Productivity (Baltimore: John Hopkins).
Kerlinger, Fred N., and Elazar J. Pedhazur. 1973. Multiple Regression in Behavioral Research (New York: Holt, Rinehart and Winston).
Kim, J., and J. Curry. 1977. The treatment of missing data in multivariate analysis, Sociological Methods Res. 6:215-240.
Kim, Jae-On. 1975. Multivariate analysis of ordinal variables, Am. J. Sociol. 88:261-298.
______ and Charles W. Mueller. 1976. Standardized and unstandardized coefficients in causal analysis, Sociological Methods and Research 4:423-438.
_______. 1978. Factor Analysis: Statistical Methods and Practical Issues (Beverly Hills, Ca.: Sage Publications).
_______. 1978. Introduction to Factor Analysis (Beverly Hills, Ca.: Sage Publications).
Knoke, D. 1975. A comparison of log-linear and regression models for systems of dichotomous variables, Sociological Methods and Research 3:416-434.
Knowles, M.C. 1964. A review of labor turnover research, Personnel Practice Bull. 20:25-37.
Kramer, Marlene. 1968. Nurse role deprivation: A symptom of needed change, Social Sci. Med. 2:461-474.
________. 1969. Collegiate graduate nurses in medical center hospitals: Mutual challenge or duel, Nursing Res. 18:196-210.
________. 1974. Reality Shock (St. Louis: Mosby).
________, and Constance Baker. 1971. The exodus: Can we prevent it? J. Nursing Admin. 1:15-30.
Kraut, A.I. 1975. Predicting turnover of employees from measured job attitudes, Organizational Behavior and Human Performance 13:233-243.
Labovitz, Sanford. 1967. Some observations on measurement and statistics, Social Forces 28:151-160.
________. 1970. The assignment of numbers to rank order categories, Am. Sociol. Rev. 35:515-524.
Ladinsky, Jack. 1967. Occupational determinants of geographic mobility among professional workers, Am. Sociol. Rev. 32:257-264.
Land, Kenneth C. 1969. Principles of path analysis, Sociological Methodology, ed. Edgar F. Borgatta (San Francisco: Jossey-Bass).
Larson, Magali Sarfatti. 1977. The Rise of Professionalism (Berkeley: Univ. of California Press).
Lawler, Edward E. 1971. Pay and Organizational Effectiveness (New York: McGraw-Hill).
________. 1973. Motivation in Work Organizations (Monterey; Ca.: Brooks/Cole).
Lawrence, Paul, and Jay Lorsch. 1969. Organization and Environment (Homewood; Ill.: Irwin).
Lazarsfeld, Paul F. 1959. Problems in methodology, Sociology Today: Problems and Prospects, eds. Robert K. Merton, Leonard Broom, and Leonard S. Cottrell, Jr. (New York: Harper and Row).
Lefkowitz, Joel. 1971. Personnel turnover, Progress in Clinical Psychology, ed. L.E. Abt and B.F. Reiss (New York: Grune and Stratton).

_______ and Myron L. Katz. 1969. Validity of exit interviews, Personnel Psychol. 22:445-455.
Leslie, G., and A.H. Richardson. 1961. Life cycle, career pattern, and the decision to move, Am. Sociol. Rev. 26:894-902.
Levine, Eugene, and Stuart Wright. 1957. New ways to measure personnel turnover in hospitals, Hospitals 31:38-42.
Lindenfeld, Frank. 1963. Teacher Turnover in Public Elementary and Secondary Schools, 1959-1960 (Washington, D.C.: U.S. Government Printing Office).
Lipset, Seymour M. 1963. The First New Nation (New York: Basic Books).
Locke, Edwin A. 1976. The nature and causes of job satisfaction, Handbook of Industrial and Organizational Psychology, ed. Marvin D. Dunnette (Chicago: Rand McNally).
Long, L.H. 1972. The influence of number and ages of children on residential mobility, Demography 9:371-382.
Longbein, Laura I., and Allan J. Lichtman. 1978. Ecological Inference (Beverly Hills, Ca.: Sage Publications).
Lyons, Thomas F. 1968. Nursing Attitudes and Turnover (Ames: Industrial Relations Center, Iowa State Univ.).
_______. 1970. Reducing nursing turnover, Hospitals 44:74-80.
Lysaught, Jerome P. 1970. An Abstract for Action (New York: McGraw-Hill).
McGee, Reece. 1971. Academic Janus (San Francisco: Jossey-Bass).
Mangione, Thomas W. 1973. Turnover-Some psychological and demographic correlates, The 1969-1970 Survey of Working Conditions, ed. Robert P. Quinn and Thomas W. Mangione (Ann Arbor: Final Report to Employment Standards Administration, U.S. Department of Labor, Survey Research Center, Univ. of Micigan).
March, James G., and Herbert A. Simon. 1958. Organizations (New York: Wiley).
Marsh, Robert M., and Hiroshi Mannari. 1971. Lifetime commitment in Japan: Roles, norms, and values, Am. J. Sociol. 76:795-812.
_______. 1972. A new look at "lifetime commitment" in Japanese industry, Econ. Develop. Cult. Change 20:611-630.
Martin, Thomas N. 1977. A structural analysis of the determinants of voluntary turnover (unpublished Ph.D. dissertation, Univ. of Iowa).
Mason, Ward S., and Robert K. Bain. 1959. Teacher Turnover in the Public Schools, 1957-1958 (Washington, D.C.: U.S. Government Printing Office).
Mattila, J. Peter. 1974. Job quitting and frictional unemployment, Am. Econ. Rev. 64:235-239.
Mauksch, Hans O. 1957. Nursing dilemmas in the organization of patient care, Nursing Outlook 5:31-33.
_______. 1965. The nurse: Coordinator of patient care, Social Interaction and Patient Care, ed. J.K. Skipper, Jr. and R.C. Leonard (Philadelphia: J.B. Lippincott).
Mayo, Elton. 1924. Revery and industrial fatigue, Personnel J. 8:273-281.
_______ and George F.F. Lombard. 1944. Teamwork and Labor Turnover in the Aircraft Industry of Southern California (Boston: Graduate School of Business Administration, Harvard Univ.).
Melbin, Murray, and Doris L. Taub. 1966. The high cost of replacing a nurse, Hospitals 40:112-122.
Merton, Robert K. 1957. Social Theory and Social Structure (New York: Free Press).
Miller, Sheila J. 1976. Family life cycle, extended family orientations, and economic aspirations as factors in the propensity to migrate, Sociological Quart. 17:323-335.

Mobley, William H. 1977. Intermediate linkages in the relationship between job satisfaction and employee turnover, J. Appl. Psychol. 62:237-240.

_______, Herbert H. Hand, Robert L. Baker, and Bruce M. Meglino. 1979a. Conceptual and empirical analysis of military recruit training attrition, J. Appl. Psychol. 64:10-18.

_______, R.W. Griffeth, H.H. Hand, and B.M. Meglino. 1979b. Review and conceptual analysis of the employee turnover process, Psychological Bull. 86:493-522.

Mobley, William H., Stanley O. Horner, and A.T. Hollingsworth. 1978. An evaluation of precursors of hospital employee turnover, J. Appl. Psychol. 63:408-414.

Moffatt, G.W.B., and Kate Hill. 1970. Labour turnover in Australia-A review of research, Part I, Personnel Practice Bull. 26:142-149.

Mosteller, F., and D.P. Moynihan. 1972. On Equality of Educational Opportunity (New York: Random House).

Mowday, Richard T., Richard M. Steers, and Lyman W. Porter. 1979. The measurement of organizational commitment, J. Vocational Behav. 14:224-247.

Muchinsky, Paul M., and Mark L. Tuttle. 1979. Employee turnover: An empirical and methodological assessment, J. Vocational Behav. 14:43-77.

National Opinion Research Center (Andrew M. Greeley and Richard A. Schoenherr, co-investigators). 1972. The Catholic Priest in the United States (Washington, D.C.: U.S. Catholic Conference).

Nunnally, J.C. 1967. Psychometric Theory (New York: McGraw-Hill).

Organization for Economic Cooperation and Development. 1965. Wages and Labor Mobility (Paris: Organization for Economic Cooperation and Development).

Parsons, Donald O. 1972. Specific human capital: An application to quit rates and layoff rates, J. Political Econ. 80:1120-1143.

_______. 1973. Quit rates over time: A search and information approach, Am. Econ. Rev. 63:390-401.

Parsons, Talcott. 1949. The Structure of Social Action (New York: Free Press).

Pencavel, John H. 1970. An Analysis of the Quite Rate in American Manufacturing Industry (Princeton; N.J.: Industrial Relations Section, Department of Economics, Princeton Univ.).

_______. 1972. Wages, specific training and labor turnover in U.S. manufacturing industries, Intern. Econ. Rev. 13:53-64.

Perrow, Charles. 1967. A framework for the comparative analysis of organizations, Am. Sociol. Rev. 32:194-208.

Peterson, Robert W., and Richard A. Schoenherr. 1978. Organizational status attainment of religious professionals, Social Forces 50:794-822.

Pettman, B.O. 1973. Some factors influencing labor turnover: A review of reserach literature, Ind. Relations 4:43-61.

Pfeffer, Jeffrey, and Gerald R. Salancik. 1978. The External Control of Organizations (New York: Harper & Row).

Porter, Lyman W., and Richard M. Steers. 1973. Organizational, work, and personal factors in employee turnover and absenteeism, Psychological Bull. 80:151-176.

Price, James L. 1968. Organizational Effectiveness (Homewood; Ill.: Irwin).

_______. 1972a. Handbook of Organizational Measurement (Lexington; Ma.: D.C. Heath).

_______. 1972b. The study of organizational effectiveness, Sociological Quart. 13:3-15.

_______. 1977. The Study of Turnover (Ames: Iowa State Univ. Press).

________, and Allen C. Bluedorn. 1979. Test of a causal model of turnover from organizations, The International Yearbook of Organizational Studies, ed. D. Dunkerley and G. Salaman (London: Routledge and Kegan Paul).

Rice, A.K. 1953. An approach to problems of labor turnover: A case study, Brit. Management Rev. 2:19-47.

Riley, Matilda W. 1964. Sources and types of sociological data, Handbook of Modern Sociology, ed. R.E.L. Faris (Chicago: Rand-McNally).

Robinson, W.S. 1950. Ecological correlations and the behavior of individuals, Am. Sociol. Rev. 15:351-357.

Ronan, W.W. 1967. A study of some concepts concerning labor turnover, Occupational Psychol. 41:193-200.

Rosenberg, Morris. 1968. The Logic of Survey Analysis (New York: Basic Books).

Ross, Arthur M. 1958. Do we have a new industrial feudalism? Am. Econ. Rev. 48:903-920.

Russell, J. D. 1968. Labour turnover and absence: Effect of location and size of undertaking, Personnel Practice Bull. 24:28-36.

Salancik, G.R. 1977. Commitment and the control of organizational behavior and belief, New Directions in Organizational Behavior, ed. B.M. Staw and G.R. Salancik (Chicago: St. Clair Press).

Schoenherr, Richard A., and Andrew M. Greeley. 1974. Role commitment process and the American Catholic priesthood, Am. Sociol. Rev. 39: 407-426.

Schoonhoven, Claudia B. 1977. Problems with the contingency theory: An empirical test of assumptions hidden within the language of contingency theory. Paper, American Sociological Association, Chicago.

Schuh, Allen J. 1967. The predictability of employee tenure: A review of the literature, Personnel Psychol. 20:133-152.

Scott, Richard D. 1972. Job expectancy-an important factor in labor turnover, Personnel J. 51:360-363.

Sloan, Frank A. 1975. The Geographic Distribution of Nurses & Public Policy (Bethesda, Md.: U.S. Department of Health, Education, and Welfare, Bureau of Health Manpower, Division of Nursing).

________. 1978. Equalizing Access to Nursing Services: The Geographic Dimension (Hyattsville, Md.: U.S. Department of Health, Education, and Welfare, Bureau of Health Manpower, Division of Nursing).

Smith, F.J., and W.A. Kerr. 1953. Turnover factors as assessed by the exit interview, J. Appl. Psychol. 37:352-355.

Smith, Patricia C., Lorne M. Kendall, and Charles L. Hulin. 1969. The Measurement of Satisfaction in Work and Retirement (Chicago: Rand McNally).

Stapleton, David C. 1977. Analyzing political participation data with a MIMIC model, Sociological Methodology 1978, ed. Karl F. Schuessler (San Francisco: Jossey-Bass).

Stoikov, Vladimir, and Robert L. Raimon. 1968. Determinants of differences in the quit rate among industries, Am. Econ. Rev. 58:1283-1298.

Stolzenberg, Ross M. 1975. Occupations labor markets and the process of wage attainment, Am. Sociol. Rev. 40:645-665.

Survey Research Center. 1975. The Michigan Organizational Assessment Package (Ann Arbor, Mich.: Institute of Social Research).

Taino, Risto. 1977. Research on the Factors Associated with the Propensity to Stay in an Organization (Helsingin Kauppakorkeakoulun Julkaisuja, B-18).

Telly, Charles S., Wendell L. French, and William G. Scott. 1971. The relationship of inequity to turnover among hourly workers, Admin. Sci. Quart. 16:164-172.

Tollen, William B. 1960. Study of Staff Losses in Child Welfare and Family Service Agencies (Washington, D.C.: U.S. Government Printing Office).

U.S. Bureau of the Census. 1970. Census of Population: 1970. General Social and Economic Characteristics. Final Report PC(1). U.S. Department of Commerce.

U.S. Bureau of the Census. 1975. Statistical Abstract of the United States. U.S. Department of Commerce.

U.S. Bureau of Labor Statistics. 1975. Handbook of Labor Statistics (Washington, D.C.: U.S. Government Printing Office).

U.S. Children's Bureau, Child Welfare Statistics, 1964, HEW Stat. Ser. 82, 1965.

U.S. National Center for Health Statistics. 1976. Health Resources Statistics. U.S. Department of Health

Valenzi, E.R., and I.R. Andrews. 1971. Effects of hourly overpay and underpay inequity when tested with a new induction procedure, J. Appl. Psychol. 55:22-27.

Van der Merwe, Roux, and Sylvia Miller. 1970. Labor Turnover in the South African Footwear Industry (Grahamston: Leather Industries Research Institute Res. Bull. 535).

________. 1971. The measurement of labor turnover, Human Relations 24:233-253.

________. 1973. Near-terminal labor turnover: An analysis of a crisis situation, Human Relations 26:415-432.

________. 1976. Measuring Absence and Labor Turnover (Johannesburg, S.A.: McGraw-Hill).

Vroom, Victor H. 1964. Work and Motivation (New York: Wiley).

Wanous, John P. 1973. Effects of a realistic preview on job acceptance, job attitudes, and job survival, J. Appl. Psychol. 58:327-332.

Wattenberg, Ben J., and Richard M. Scammon. 1965. This U.S.A.: An Unexpected Family Portrait of 194,067,296 Americans Drawn from the Census (Garden City, N.Y.: Doubleday).

Whyte, William H., Jr. 1956. The Organization Man (New York: Simon & Schuster).

Wieland, George F. 1969. Studying and measuring nursing turnover, Int. J. Nursing Studies 6:61-70.

Wilensky, Harold. 1964. The professionalization of everyone? Am. J. Sociol. 70:137-158.

Woodward, Joan. 1965. Industrial Organization: Theory and Practice (London: Oxford University Press).

Wright, James D., and Richard F. Hamilton. 1978. Work satisfaction and age: Some evidence for the job change hypothesis, Social Forces 56: 1140-1158.

Zetterberg, Hans L. 1965. On Theory and Verification in Sociology (Totowa, New Jersey: Bedminster).

Index